Fast Facts

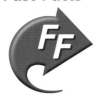

D1316868

Multiple Sclerosis

Second edition

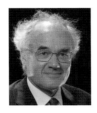

George D Perkin BA FRCP
Consultant Neurologist
West London Neurosciences Centre
The Hammersmith Hospitals NHS Trust
London, UK

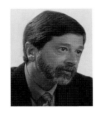

Jerry S Wolinsky MD
Bartels Family and Opal C Rankin Professor of Neurology
The University of Texas
Health Science Center at Houston
Houston, Texas, USA

Declaration of Independence
This book is as balanced and as practical as we can make it.
Ideas for improvement are always welcome:
feedback@fastfacts.com

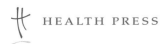

HEALTH PRESS

Fast Facts: Multiple Sclerosis
First published 2000
Second edition January 2006

Text © 2006 George D Perkin, Jerry S Wolinsky
© 2006 in this edition Health Press Limited
Health Press Limited, Elizabeth House, Queen Street, Abingdon,
Oxford OX14 3LN, UK
Tel: +44 (0)1235 523233
Fax: +44 (0)1235 523238

Book orders can be placed by telephone or via the website.
For regional distributors or to order via the website, please go to:
www.fastfacts.com
For telephone orders, please call 01752 202301 (UK), +44 1752 202301 (Europe),
1 800 247 6553 (USA, toll free) or +1 419 281 1802 (Americas).

Fast Facts is a trademark of Health Press Limited.

A CIP record for this title is available from the British Library.

ISBN 1-903734-70-3

Perkin GD (George)
Fast Facts: Multiple Sclerosis/
George D Perkin, Jerry S Wolinsky

Medical illustrations by Annamaria Dutto, Withernsea, UK.
Typesetting and page layout by Zed, Oxford, UK.
Printed by Fine Print (Services) Ltd, Oxford, UK.

Printed with vegetable inks on fully biodegradable and
recyclable paper manufactured from sustainable forests.

444   001
Low emissions
during production

Low   Sustainable
chlorine   forests

Introduction

Until relatively recently, the diagnosis of multiple sclerosis (MS) was often subject to error. The advent of magnetic resonance imaging (MRI) made more accurate diagnosis possible, and for the first time it became possible to recognize the very early stages of the disease. In 2001, the International Panel on the Diagnosis of Multiple Sclerosis, chaired by Professor WI McDonald of the Royal College of Physicians, London, issued new diagnostic criteria that integrated the use of MRI findings to ensure rapid and accurate diagnosis of the disease. These criteria have recently undergone further review and revision, and are discussed in detail in Chapter 4.

Previously, the treatment of MS was largely confined to short-term injections or steroid tablets, alongside symptomatic measures. Now, the availability of interferon drugs and glatiramer acetate has enabled clinicians to alter the long-term natural history of the disease. Early data on natalizumab clearly indicate that an expanding armamentarium of more effective immunomodulatory agents based on the principles of molecular biology is on the way; however, such data also underscore the potential risks that immune manipulation may bring. This book gives a revised overview of the immunomodulatory drugs that reduce the risk of future attacks and may also slow the rate of acquisition of neurological dysfunction. It also covers steroid therapy for acute attacks and the range of treatments available for symptoms associated with the disease. There is updated information on pain management and discussion of the latest evidence on the role of cannabinoids.

The book examines the importance of a multidisciplinary team approach in providing MS patients with the best possible quality of life. Case histories punctuate the text and explore the lessons that can be learned from the experiences of patients coping with the disease.

We hope that this second edition of *Fast Facts: Multiple Sclerosis* will be a useful guide for all healthcare professionals working with patients who have this complex disease.

Epidemiology, pathology and pathophysiology

Multiple sclerosis (MS) is characterized by recurrent or chronically progressive neurological dysfunction. It is caused by perivenular inflammatory foci in the white matter of the central nervous system (CNS). Repeated episodes of inflammation result in characteristic widespread, demyelinated and sclerotic lesions, referred to as plaques, throughout the brain, optic nerves and spinal cord of affected individuals. An immune-mediated component is central to disease pathogenesis.

Epidemiology

MS is the most common non-traumatic, disabling neurological disease in young adults. Overall, the prevalence is about 100 cases per 100 000 people. This amounts to about 350 000 cases in the USA and Canada, and an almost equal number of cases in Europe, including the UK. However, the incidence of the disease varies markedly according to age, sex, location and genetic background.

Age, sex and ethnic origin. The age of onset peaks at about 30 years, with fewer than 10% of all cases starting before puberty or after the age of 55 years. Women are disproportionately represented in all patient series, with a ratio of about 2:1. White populations, particularly people of Scandinavian ancestry, have a high risk of the disease, though few ethnic groups are spared.

Geographic distribution. The disease shows a geographic gradient of prevalence, with more cases found at the northern latitudes of Europe and North America and at the southern latitudes of New Zealand and Australia (Figure 1.1). This variation strongly suggests the involvement of environmental factors in the pathogenesis of the disease. Despite research into possible environmental triggers, such as viral or bacterial infections, toxins, duration of sunlight, changes

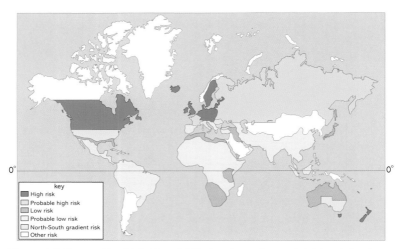

Figure 1.1 Geographic distribution of MS, showing patterns of risk in relation to region of residence. Areas of high risk are found at high latitudes. Reprinted from McAlpine et al. *Multiple Sclerosis: A Reappraisal*, 1965. Edinburgh: Livingstone. Copyright 1965, with permission from Elsevier.

in temperature and humidity, and diet, no specific environmental factor has been shown to cause MS.

Migration studies have shown that the risk of developing the disease can be attributed to the region of childhood residence. For example, it appears that an individual born in a high-risk area can acquire a lower risk if they relocate to a low-risk area before they reach 15 years of age. Reports of apparent disease epidemics in specific areas further support the hypothesis for a geographic influence on the disease.

Genetic factors. While increased MS risk is conferred by the *DRB1*1501 (DR2)* haplotype of the major histocompatibility complex, multiple genetic loci are likely to contribute interactively to the risk. Human leukocyte antigen (HLA)-DR molecules are critical in the immune system, where they present and process both foreign and self-antigens.

Table 1.1 gives an overview of the familial risk of the disease, which may be helpful when counseling family members of newly

TABLE 1.1

Age-adjusted risks of familial MS

Relationship to index case	Male index (%)	Female index (%)
Parent	2.6	3.0
Child	2.5	2.6
Sibling	3.8	4.0
First cousin	1.5	2.4

Data from Sadovnick AD et al. *Am J Med Genet* 1988;29:533–41.

diagnosed patients. The overall risk of the disease is about 1 per 1000 individuals when there is no familial history of MS, but it increases by a factor of 10–20 if there are known relatives with the disease. Moreover, studies in twins from different populations consistently indicate that a monozygotic twin of an MS patient is at higher risk (25–30% concordance) for MS than is a dizygotic twin (2–5%).

Pathology

Plaques are the hallmark pathology of MS, and can occur at any site where there are myelinated axons within the CNS. Myelin is a complex extension of the cytoplasmic membranes of oligodendroglial cells, which cover the large-diameter axons of the CNS.

Myelinated axons are able to conduct impulses rapidly. High rates of conduction are necessary for successful transfer of information between neurons to allow coordinated motor movements, as well as sensory perception and facile cognition.

Most often, plaques are found in the:
- periventricular region of the brain
- optic nerves
- spinal cord
- subcortical white matter of the cerebral hemispheres
- cerebral cortex (involved in most cases).

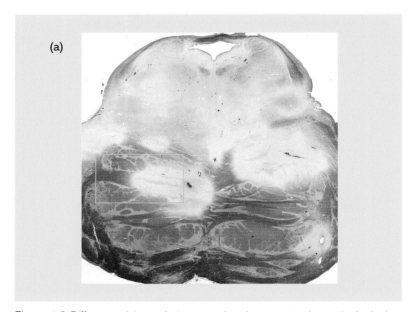

Figure 1.2 Different staining techniques used to demonstrate plaques in the brain of a patient with MS. (a) A section through the pons at the level of the third-nerve nuclei stained specifically for myelin (black). Multiple ovoid areas fail to stain, reflecting the presence of well-developed MS plaques. The region within the yellow box is shown in detail on the opposite page, and arrows highlight the same region of crossing fibers in the pons. (b) A section stained with hematoxylin and eosin; the crossing fibers are pale as they enter the edge of the plaque. (c) A section stained for myelin: there is a loss of staining for the same fibers entering the plaque. (d) An axonal silver stain; it is difficult to determine where the plaque is located because of the relative sparing of axons.

Plaques in the pons region of the brain are shown in Figure 1.2. Distribution of the lesions varies considerably from case to case, mirroring in part the varied clinical presentations of the disease.

Individual plaques show variable amounts of perivenular and parenchymal mononuclear-cell inflammation, demyelination with relative axonal sparing, oligodendroglial cell loss and astrocytic proliferation with gliosis (Figure 1.3).

Several stages of lesion formation probably exist, and plaques are characterized as acute, subacute or chronic.

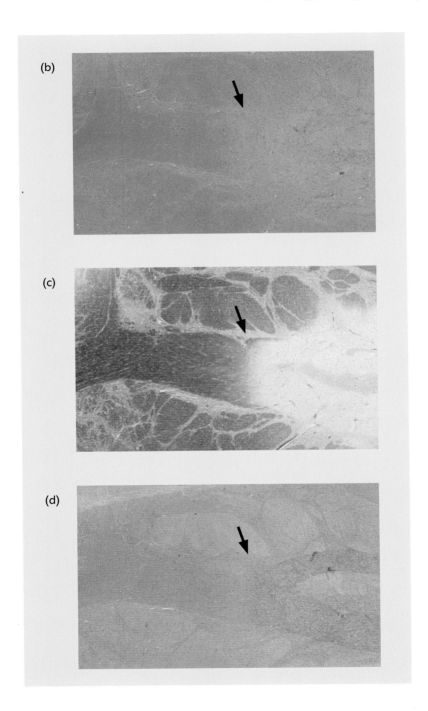

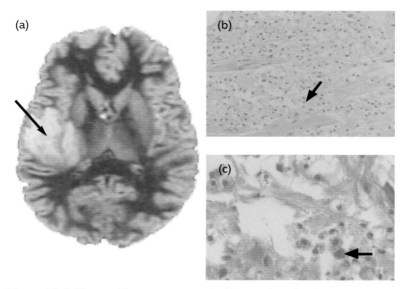

Figure 1.3 A 32-year-old woman presented with several weeks of progressive left-sided numbness. (a) A dual-inversion recovery MRI scan disclosed a large lesion (see arrow), restricted to the white matter of the right temporal-parietal region; normal white matter and CSF appear dark, and gray matter structures appear light gray. A cerebral biopsy was performed to obtain a definitive diagnosis and eliminate the possibility of a tumor. (b) Tissue staining with hematoxylin and eosin disclosed a sea of macrophages separated by strands of cytoplasm of reactive astrocytes (arrowed). (c) Staining with Luxol fast blue showed that macrophage cytoplasm contained recently degraded myelin, stained purple (arrowed). Staining for axons displayed their relative preservation in the biopsy material (not shown). A few small high-signal-intensity lesions were found in the white matter of the opposite hemisphere, and examination of CSF disclosed 47 lymphocytes, an increased rate of synthesis of immunoglobulin G and a single oligoclonal band. The patient's symptoms resolved following treatment with intravenous methylprednisolone, and she responded well to interferon therapy. Massive demyelinating lesions of this type are uncommon and, when solitary, they mimic tumors and may have a monophasic disease course.

In white matter, a perivascular infiltrate of T cells and macrophages initially predominates. The vascular endothelium, which normally acts as a barrier to many bloodborne molecules entering the brain, becomes inflamed and expresses a number of molecules that attract additional cells (see Lesion formation, page 14). In areas where the endothelium is focally disrupted, the myelin is engulfed by macrophages and actively degraded. Numerous macrophages are found that contain the products of myelin breakdown, including myelin proteins and lipids. Some oligodendrocytes persist, and these may attempt to remyelinate neighboring demyelinated axons. However, most oligodendrocytes within these lesions show cytolytic changes and die. Astrocytes are activated. Some demyelinated axons are transected, and are unable to re-establish distant connections, leading to irreversible neurological dysfunction. Chronic lesions show little inflammation, an absence of oligodendroglial cells (except at their extreme margins) and an intense astrogliosis. In some chronic lesions, axonal loss can be marked.

Pathophysiology

Axon function. Electrical conduction and signal transmission along the larger axons of the CNS are facilitated by the formation of internodes, which have a high concentration of sodium channels, along the axon. The internodal regions are separated by heavily myelinated segments. During MS attacks, impulse transmission fails across demyelinated axon segments; this failure causes the associated symptoms. Conduction is restored by remyelination, which re-establishes a near-normal internodal architecture; the clinical attack subsequently regresses. However, the factors that contribute to conduction block and the restoration of effective, if not normal, conduction are more complicated than this simple construct. Other factors likely to influence the loss and return of clinical function in the face of chronic demyelination include:

- neuroelectrical blocking factors in serum
- reorganization of sodium channels along demyelinated nodes
- release of nitric oxide from inflammatory cells
- activated microglia.

Axonal loss (when axons are transected) is highly correlated with non-reversible neurological impairment.

13

Lesion formation. Some of the events that contribute to lesion formation are now reasonably well understood. During the course of any viral infection, macrophages take up the viral proteins and degrade them into their individual antigenic components. The antigens are presented as protein fragments on the surfaces of macrophages by their HLA-DR molecules, and are recognized by the immune system.

Normally, the presentation of these antigens to the immune system leads to the activation of T cells, which begins a cascade that results in elimination of the virus. However, in MS, it is postulated that a portion of the responding cells mistakes the viral antigen for a self-protein, probably a protein found in myelin.

The number of systemically activated effector T cells (pro-inflammatory CD4+ T helper [Th]1 cells) increases in the circulation. These cells then enter the brain at sites with an increased display of surface adhesion molecules on the vascular endothelium to cause further disruption of the blood–brain barrier. Although adhesion molecules occur normally on the endothelium, they increase in number when the endothelium is damaged, then attract T cells and help them to enter the brain.

As the T cells migrate into the brain and encounter myelin antigens, they secrete a number of chemokines and cytokines, namely interleukin-2 (IL-2), tumor necrosis factor alpha (TNFα) and interferon gamma (IFNγ) (Figure 1.4). These substances recruit antigen-non-specific mononuclear cells, thus amplifying the cascade of myelin-destructive substances in the region of the developing lesion. This intense, perivenular inflammation is associated with local disruption of the blood–brain barrier, the development of vasogenic edema and the influx of myelinotoxic substances from the blood, including certain immunoglobulins and complement factors.

Macrophages and activated microglia engulf and degrade myelin, stripping it from axons that traverse the lesion (see Figure 1.4). With intense activity, oligodendroglia are lost and axons are transected. However, in some lesions, despite active myelin breakdown, the surviving oligodendroglia can remyelinate the surviving demyelinated axons.

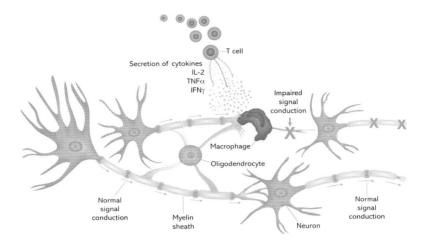

Figure 1.4 Proposed model of an immune-mediated attack on the myelin sheath of an axon, in which the neuron has been partially demyelinated. The neuron is surrounded by T cells, which secrete inflammatory cytokines and chemokines (IFNγ, interferon gamma; IL-2, interleukin-2; TNFα, tumor necrosis factor alpha), and by macrophages, which strip the myelin from the axon, resulting in demyelination and consequent impairment of signal conduction.

It is likely that another type of T cell, CD4+ Th2, which secretes regulatory cytokines interleukin-4 (IL-4) and transforming growth factor beta (TGFβ), eventually suppresses the inflammatory response and limits damage. Major changes in regional vascular permeability resolve over weeks, and the products of myelin breakdown are removed over months. As the inflammation subsides, only scant inflammatory cells, often immunoglobulin-secreting B cells, remain.

Astrocytes are activated early in lesion formation, and contribute to the intense gliosis, which is the type of scarring that occurs in the CNS and characterizes many chronic plaques. The destructive process is repeated in an unpredictable manner in previously unaffected regions of CNS white matter. It can also recur at sites of remyelination or incomplete demyelination, and can extend at the edges of chronic lesions, involving more white matter over time.

Activation of systemic, pro-inflammatory CD4+ Th1 cells can follow a variety of non-specific viral infections. These infections are the well-recognized precipitants of clinical attacks. However, the events that initiate the unregulated expansion of putative antigen-specific T cells, or trigger the influx of these cells into the brain, are unknown. Similarly, it is unclear if the immunoregulatory abnormalities that have been demonstrated repeatedly in patients with MS are primary or secondary to an abnormality in the maintenance of CNS myelin, as might be seen with a persistent viral infection.

Key points – epidemiology, pathology and pathophysiology

- The development of MS reflects a complex interplay of genes (those that predispose to disease and others that may modify the disease course), environmental triggers, disease-course modifiers and aberrant immune responses.
- Age of disease onset peaks at 30 years.
- Women are twice as likely as men to develop MS.
- Plaques are the hallmark pathology of MS. They can occur at any site within the CNS where there are myelinated axons.
- While inflammatory demyelination is the hallmark of the disease, axonal transection and neuronal loss contribute to the accumulation of irreversible clinical disability.

Key references

Bo L, Vedeler CA, Nyland H et al. Intracortical multiple sclerosis lesions are not associated with increased lymphocyte infiltration. *Mult Scler* 2003;9:323–31.

Bradl M, Hohlfeld R. Molecular pathogenesis of neuroinflammation. *J Neurol Neurosurg Psychiatry* 2003;74:1364–70.

Dyment DA, Ebers GC, Sadovnick AD. Genetics of multiple sclerosis. *Lancet Neurol* 2004;3:104–10.

Kapoor R, Davies M, Blaker PA et al. Blockers of sodium and calcium entry protect axons from nitric oxide-mediated degeneration. *Ann Neurol* 2003;53:174–80.

Lucchinetti C, Bruck W, Parisi J et al. Heterogeneity of multiple sclerosis lesions: implications for the pathogenesis of demyelination. *Ann Neurol* 2000;47:707–17.

Trapp BD, Peterson J, Ransohoff RM et al. Axonal transection in the lesions of multiple sclerosis. *N Engl J Med* 1998;338:278–85.

Wallin MT, Page WF, Kurtzke JF. Multiple sclerosis in US veterans of the Vietnam era and later military service: race, sex, and geography. *Ann Neurol* 2004;55:65–71.

Classification

The major types of multiple sclerosis (MS), based on distinctive clinical presentations, are:
- remitting relapsing disease
- secondary progressive disease
- primary progressive disease
- progressive relapsing disease.

Of these, remitting relapsing and secondary progressive are by far the most common. Primary progressive disease occurs in no more than 15% of all MS patients, and fewer than 5% of MS patients have the progressive relapsing form. While these disease subtypes can be easily described, many patients fit poorly into them. The best distinction can be made between the relapsing forms of the disease (i.e. remitting relapsing and secondary progressive) and primary progressive disease, as certain characteristics of magnetic resonance imaging (MRI) scans often differ between these two disease types. It is uncertain whether these accepted standard definitions will withstand scrutiny or lead to a better understanding of MS as a disease process.

Prodromal symptoms

The initial neurological presentation of MS may be preceded by non-specific complaints, such as fatigue, altered appetite, mood change or memory disturbance. However, as most patients attending outpatient departments tend to have such symptoms, their specificity is open to question.

Remitting relapsing disease

This is, by far, the most common form of MS. Characteristically, patients experience acute attacks of neurological dysfunction, during which new symptoms appear or existing symptoms become more severe. It is rare for the neurological symptoms and signs to develop in an apoplectic fashion. More commonly, symptoms of neurological dysfunction increase over a number of days to several weeks before reaching a maximum. If untreated, the dysfunction persists for several days or weeks before complete or incomplete recovery occurs over a period of weeks to months. Recovery from these discrete attacks or relapses is typically most rapid and most complete at disease onset.

Definition. Several definitions of the acute attack have been suggested, particularly for uniformity in the design and conduct of clinical trials. These definitions also serve the clinician well. A discrete clinical attack can be defined by the following criteria:

- new or recurrent neurological signs and symptoms lasting at least 24–48 hours
- symptoms that occur after at least 30 days of stable neurological function
- new or recurrent symptoms and signs that appear in the absence of fever, intercurrent infection or other notable metabolic derangements (MS patients may experience transient recurrence of symptoms from previous attacks if they have a fever or experience any metabolic insult)
- objective signs of neurological dysfunction that can reasonably be linked to the involvement of central myelinated pathways (such signs are required in most clinical trials).

In general, clinicians are well advised to look for this last criterion. This requirement is most readily fulfilled by objective examination when the symptoms suggest involvement of the motor, visual or coordination pathway. It can often be difficult to substantiate neurological dysfunction when the patient's symptoms are solely sensory; for example, well-reported symptoms of numbness in an arm or leg may lack objective confirmation on neurological examination, even though they may be clearly evident to the patient.

The definition of remitting relapsing disease does not require a return to normal, symptom-free neurological function following an attack. However, any residual symptoms, neurological findings or

disability acquired during an attack must remain stable between attacks. In this form of the disease, any accumulation of neurological deterioration occurs in a stepwise fashion, after well-defined acute exacerbations or relapses. These two patterns of remitting relapsing MS are visually depicted in Figure 2.1:
- relapses with a return to normal neurological function
- relapsing disease with stepwise, accumulated disability.

Presenting symptoms. Acute presenting symptoms typical of remitting relapsing MS take many forms, as described below. The incidence of initial symptoms in one series of patients is given in Table 2.1.

Weakness. An episode of heaviness in one or both lower limbs, or a complaint of exercise-induced weakness and heaviness of the lower limbs, are common presenting features in patients with MS (Case history 2.1). Examination may show little in such patients save, perhaps, depression of the abdominal reflexes or an extensor plantar response on one side. Less commonly, some patients present with acute weakness of the lower limbs with, in effect, complete cord transection; however, most of these patients do not progress to MS during a protracted follow-up period.

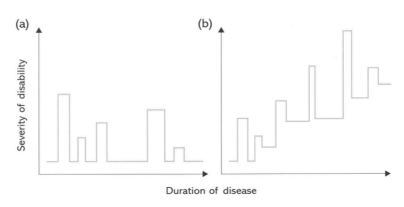

Figure 2.1 The two patterns of remitting relapsing disease: (a) relapses with return to normal neurological function; (b) relapsing disease with stepwise, accumulated disability.

TABLE 2.1

Initial symptoms in one series of patients with remitting relapsing MS

Initial symptom	Incidence (%)
Weakness	40
Loss of vision	22
Paresthesias	21
Diplopia	12
Vertigo	5
Altered micturition	5

Case history 2.1 – limb weakness

A 45-year-old woman developed a loss of reactivity in her right leg 4 months before presentation. The leg failed to respond properly when she tried to move it. It felt heavy and she began to trip. She noticed slight weakness and clumsiness of the right hand, with a loss of precision in her writing. On examination, she was found to have slightly brisker reflexes in the right arm than the left, and a minor loss of dexterity in the right hand. The patient had some weakness in the right leg, but somewhat brisker reflexes in the right leg than the left. She had flexor plantars.

MRI and subsequent history established a diagnosis of MS.

Weakness and/or heaviness of the limbs are common presenting symptoms.

Loss of vision typically occurs as part of an attack of acute optic neuritis. Most patients experience pain in or around the eye, which is usually exacerbated by eye movement. Shortly afterwards, visual loss occurs, but the degree to which this happens can vary; some patients effectively become blind in the affected eye. Findings include a field defect (predominantly central in most patients) and

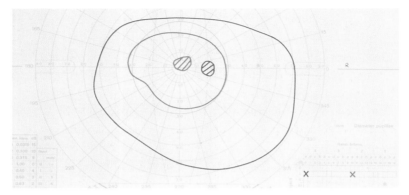

Figure 2.2 Right central scotoma in a patient with optic neuritis. The scotoma is hatched in red, the blind spot is hatched in blue.

an abnormal pupillary response to light (Figure 2.2). The optic disc may be swollen and is sometimes surrounded by hemorrhages. The majority of patients recover their vision over a median period of about 8 weeks.

Paresthesias occur in characteristic patterns that may spread from one leg to the other and then to a level on the trunk, or present as altered sensation in the periphery of one or more limbs (Case history 2.2). Objective findings may be slight, but it is worth inquiring about symptoms induced by neck flexion. Some patients, even as a presenting feature, will complain that neck flexion leads to a shower of paresthesias ('electric shocks') that radiate down the spine into the legs (Lhermitte's phenomenon). Although this symptom (which is associated with pathology in the cervical spinal cord) occurs in several conditions, its presence in a young person almost always indicates MS, provided cervical trauma has been excluded.

Diplopia may develop as an isolated symptom at the onset of MS, or be part of a more global disturbance of brainstem function. Sometimes abducens palsy is responsible. Isolated palsies of the third cranial nerve are uncommon in MS, and those of the fourth cranial nerve are virtually unknown. Some patients with diplopia have evidence of an internuclear ophthalmoplegia, though more commonly they describe an ill-defined blurring of vision or a

Case history 2.2 – paresthesias

A 23-year-old woman awoke 12 days before consultation with itching sensations in both hands, followed by an awareness of loss of temperature sensitivity in the right hand only. Later, the loss of temperature sensitivity spread to the right shoulder, trunk and parts of the right leg. Examination revealed loss of pain and temperature sensation on the right side, to about the C5 level. The sacral dermatomes were spared. Examination of CSF yielded normal findings. The patient recovered over 6 weeks. Four years later, the patient developed altered sensation in her legs and on the right side of her face. On examination, the findings were compatible with a fresh disturbance of the sensory pathways.

Paresthesias occur in characteristic patterns that may spread from the limbs to the trunk.

problem with visual tracking. If such patients are asked to refix their gaze between two objects in the horizontal plane, the adducting eye is seen to lag behind the abducting eye. The latter eye usually shows a few beats of nystagmus. The problem may affect the patient's gaze to one or both sides. In young people, this physical sign is almost pathognomonic of MS. Skew deviation on vertical gaze is a recognized feature (Figure 2.3).

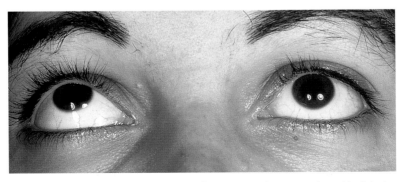

Figure 2.3 Impaired vertical gaze in the left eye in a patient presenting with diplopia.

Vertigo. In young people, vertigo is far more likely to be associated with a disorder of the vestibular apparatus in the inner ear than its central connections. If vertigo is triggered by head movement, the accompanying nystagmus tends not to fatigue and is triggered by movements in different directions, thereby distinguishing it from benign positional vertigo; in such cases, a central lesion becomes likely. In most patients, additional symptoms, such as diplopia or facial numbness, are likely to signal the origin of the symptom.

Altered micturition. Although most MS patients have altered micturition by the time the disease is fully developed, it is unusual for disturbed sphincter control to be an early feature. Symptoms include hesitancy or urgency or a mixture of both (see Sphincter function, page 38) (Case history 2.3). Disturbance of bowel control is rare in the early stages.

Symptoms triggered by certain activities. One-third of patients with fully developed MS will describe a transient exacerbation of their symptoms triggered by certain activities, particularly walking and hot baths (Uhthoff's phenomenon; Case history 2.4). This short-term exacerbation of symptoms is due to conduction in partly

---

Case history 2.3 – altered micturition

A 33-year-old woman had a 2-week history of ill-defined back pain and slight numbness in her legs. For 2 days, she had had difficulty with micturition, leading to urinary retention, for which she underwent catheterization. Bowel function and vaginal, urethral and buttock sensation were normal. Examination showed depressed abdominal responses, just-detectable spasticity of the lower limbs and bilateral extensor plantar responses. MRI showed signal changes compatible with MS. The patient received a course of corticosteroids and recovered over a period of 3 months.

Although disturbed sphincter control is unusual in the early stages of MS, symptoms may include hesitancy or urgency or both.

Case history 2.4 – Uhthoff's phenomenon

For a year, a 27-year-old man had noticed visual blurring when walking, the left eye being more affected than the right. His eyesight recovered after resting for about 30 minutes. He experienced the same problem, accompanied by weakness and unsteadiness of the legs, when he took a hot bath. On examination, the patient had left optic disc pallor and bilateral spasticity of the lower limbs with extensor plantar responses. Investigations established a diagnosis of MS.

An exacerbation of symptoms may be triggered by certain activities, such as taking a hot bath.

---

demyelinated nerve fibers in the relevant fiber pathway being blocked when body temperature rises. In some patients, exercise-induced symptoms are the first manifestation of the disease; symptoms appear during exercise and are rapidly relieved by rest. Patients with this particular presentation tend to have primary progressive MS (see page 28) rather than a remitting relapsing form of the disease.

Paroxysmal symptoms may appear during the course of the disease or at the outset (Table 2.2). Trigeminal neuralgia in MS patients cannot be distinguished from the type of neuralgia that occurs in elderly subjects, except that bilateral symptoms are more likely in MS. The neuralgia is believed to be triggered in most cases by MS lesions in the pons, close to the entry zone of the trigeminal

TABLE 2.2

Paroxysmal symptoms

- Trigeminal neuralgia
- Dysarthria and ataxia
- Tonic seizures
- Paresthesias
- Pain
- Itching

nerve; however, in some patients, as is usual with older subjects, the neuralgia appears to be due to cross-compression by blood vessels in the posterior fossa.

All paroxysmal symptoms are characterized by:
- frequency (e.g. up to 100 attacks per day)
- stereotyped nature
- brevity (seconds)
- response to carbamazepine.

After a period of days or weeks, but seldom longer, the episodes remit.

Rarer presentations in the early stages of MS include:
- altered intellectual function
- mood disturbance
- epilepsy
- symptoms that mimic a brain tumor.

Altered intellectual function is well recognized in MS, particularly in its later stages. A subcortical dementia has been described, characterized by a slowing of information processing, but with little or no evidence of cortical features, such as aphasia, apraxia or agnosia. Rarely, dementia may be prominent at the outset.

Mood disturbance is common later in the disease course, and is far more likely to manifest as depression than euphoria. However, there is no firm evidence that such problems are an initial feature of the disease.

Epilepsy is more common in MS patients than in controls, but seldom appears at the outset.

Symptoms that mimic a brain tumor are recognized features of the disease. They include a rapidly evolving hemiparesis or dysphasia, accompanied by headache. Computed tomography (CT) or MRI scans, particularly the former, may increase the confusion by showing a ring-enhancing lesion (Figure 2.4).

Progression. About 30% of MS patients will still be classified as having remitting relapsing disease 25 years after initial diagnosis. About two-thirds of patients with this disease type will have limited accumulated neurological findings and little actual disability, and

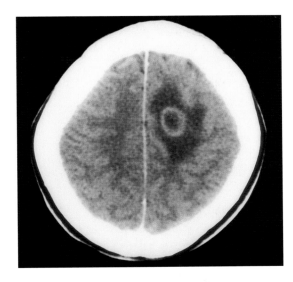

Figure 2.4
A CT scan showing
a ring-enhancing
lesion in a patient
with MS.

can be considered to have benign disease, a form of MS that cannot
be prospectively defined. Other patients with remitting relapsing
disease will eventually develop secondary progressive MS.

Secondary progressive disease

This form of MS invariably evolves from the remitting relapsing
disease type. Here, neurological disability accumulates over time,
with or without continued superimposed acute relapses (Figure 2.5).

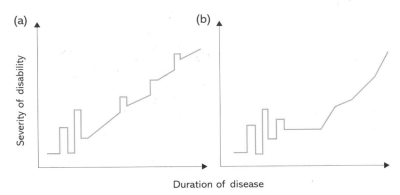

Figure 2.5 In secondary progressive MS, patients (a) may or (b) may not
continue to have relapses.

Definition. The following aspects are critical to the definition of secondary progressive disease:

- well-documented or well-recalled acute attacks of MS before entering a phase of accumulated disability
- gradual or accelerated accumulation of symptoms, neurological signs and disability from the disease in the absence of attacks, or between well-delineated relapses.

Patients who enter the secondary progressive phase of disease may or may not continue to have relapses.

Progression. Large clinical series of untreated MS patients suggest that about half of all patients will develop the secondary progressive form of the disease within 7–9 years of diagnosis. Nearly 70% of all patients with MS eventually enter a progressive phase of illness.

Primary progressive disease

This form of the disease is characterized by slowly accumulating neurological disability without prior or current well-defined attacks of neurological dysfunction (Figure 2.6).

Definition. Patients with this form of the disease often present with symptoms that suggest progressive dysfunction of the spinal cord

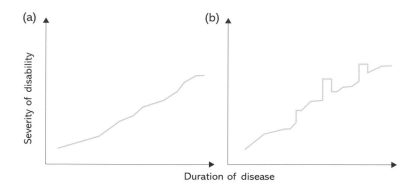

Figure 2.6 Typical patterns of disease in (a) primary progressive and (b) progressive relapsing MS.

with lower-limb weakness, tightness and reduced gait endurance. They commonly have urinary frequency and urgency.

Sometimes, when a careful history is taken of a patient with a progressive presentation, they may recall an isolated episode of neurological dysfunction, such as optic neuritis, that may have preceded the development of progressive neurological disability by one or more decades. Often, these patients have not sought medical attention for the remote symptoms, or a definite diagnosis has never been reached. By strict definition, such individuals have secondary progressive MS.

While young women tend to present with relapsing forms of the disease, men and older women are more likely to present with progressive disease from the onset. In this latter group, the prominence of symptoms suggestive of spinal-cord dysfunction should lead clinicians to make a careful search for conditions that cause progressive myelopathy (Case history 2.5).

Progression. Characteristically, patients with progressive disease have difficulty determining if they are worsening on a day-to-day, week-to-week or even month-to-month basis. They are usually able

---

Case history 2.5 – progressive myelopathy

Over a period of 18 months prior to consultation, a 60-year-old man had a progressive problem with walking. He described a loss of flexibility of the left leg. He found it particularly difficult to lift the leg, and he was unable to run. His hands had become clumsier. Examination showed dysarthria, poor lateral tongue movements and a spastic tetraparesis. The patient had mild upper- and lower-limb ataxia, and absent vibration sense in the feet. Further investigation established a diagnosis of MS.

Symptoms suggestive of spinal-cord dysfunction, especially in men and older women, should prompt further investigation to elucidate the cause of progressive myelopathy.

to determine worsening in relation to major milestones, such as from one year's holiday to the next. Things that a patient can no longer accomplish eventually become evident. The tempo of disease progression is usually slow but ingravescent; its course may be punctuated by intervals in which the patient appears quite stable, experiences some improvement for no clear reason or shows an accelerated deterioration of function overall.

Progressive relapsing disease
Progressive relapsing disease is an uncommon disease type, characterized by an initial course that simulates primary progression, but with one or more clearly defined, superimposed attacks that appear after the progressive disease is well established (see Figure 2.6).

Key points – classification and early presentation

- Classification of MS into different clinical subtypes is of practical value, with a proviso that some patients are difficult to place in such categories.
- A specific definition of an attack should be used in clinical practice.
- Up to 30% of MS patients experience transient worsening of symptoms due to heat or exercise.
- Most patients with remitting relapsing MS will enter a secondary progressive phase of the disease eventually.
- Patients who complain of paresthesias should be asked about symptoms induced by neck flexion. MS is suggested in young patients who experience a shower of paresthesias radiating down the spine into the legs.

Key references

Lublin FD, Reingold SC. Defining the clinical course of multiple sclerosis: results of an international survey. National Multiple Sclerosis Society (USA) Advisory Committee on Clinical Trials of New Agents in Multiple Sclerosis. *Neurology* 1996;46:907–11.

Lucchinetti CF, Bruck W, Rodriguez M, Lassmann H. Distinct patterns of multiple sclerosis pathology indicate heterogeneity in pathogenesis. *Brain Pathol* 1996;6:259–74.

Thompson AJ, Kermode AG, MacManus DG et al. Pattern of disease activity in multiple sclerosis: a clinical and magnetic resonance imaging study. *BMJ* 1990;300:631–4.

Twomey JA, Espir MLE. Paroxysmal symptoms as the first manifestation of multiple sclerosis. *J Neurol Neurosurg Psychiatry* 1980;43: 296–304.

Weinshenker BG, Bass, B, Rice GP et al. Natural history of multiple sclerosis: a geographically based study. I. Clinical course and disability. *Brain* 1989;112:133–46.

The features of established multiple sclerosis (MS) depend, to some extent, on the way in which the condition originally presented as well as its mode of progression. The disease course can be demonstrated in a visual format, in terms of the patient's disability against time, as shown in Figure 3.1.

For patients with benign MS, the established condition is, in a sense, not established at all. Even 15 or 20 years after presentation, these patients have little or no disability and little or no restriction of activity. In the UK at least, patients with benign MS seldom present themselves for medical attention.

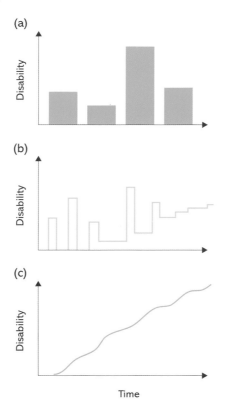

Figure 3.1 Relationship between severity of disability and duration of disease in (a) benign remitting relapsing MS, (b) remitting relapsing MS with secondary progression, and (c) primary progressive MS.

As discussed in Chapter 2, the majority of patients with MS present with a remitting relapsing form of the disease; however, many of these patients enter a secondary progressive phase, in which the frequency of relapses lessens, but residual disability emerges between attacks and then slowly progresses.

Most studies agree that relapse frequency is highest in the first few years of the disease. There is little evidence to show that relapse frequency influences outcome, but there are considerable data to indicate that the interval between the initial attack and the first relapse is significant; as this period lengthens, the likelihood of benign MS increases.

Eventually, in both primary progressive and secondary progressive MS, a fairly consistent pattern emerges, with an attendant level of disability (Figure 3.2). However, data on the disease's rate of progression and its effect on lifespan vary considerably.

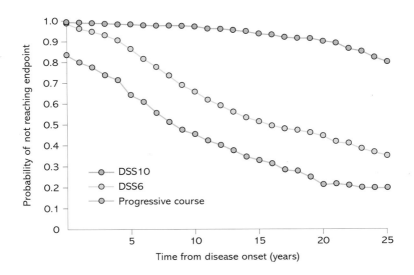

Figure 3.2 The rate at which certain endpoints are reached during the course of MS. Disability Status Score (DSS) 10, death related to the MS process; DSS 6, walking 100 m (330 ft) with assistance (e.g. with a cane or walker). Adapted from Runmarker and Andersen. 1993.

Mental function

Altered mental function is commonplace in the established condition. Indeed, studies suggest that subtle changes of intellectual function may appear quite early. In some patients, a picture of progressive intellectual impairment aligned with a gait disorder mimics the presentation of normal-pressure hydrocephalus (Case history 3.1). Depression is far more common than euphoria once the disease is established.

Visual function

After several years, many MS patients will have partial or complete pallor of one or both optic discs, regardless of whether they have had attacks of optic neuritis (Case history 3.2). This pallor reflects the combined loss of myelin, myelinated axons and vascularity of the disc. Nevertheless, visual acuity is usually preserved.

Eye movements

An internuclear ophthalmoplegia is the most common persisting oculomotor sign (other than nystagmus) in established MS. The

---

Case history 3.1 – mental impairment

A 46-year-old woman had a 4-year history of progressive cognitive impairment associated with a gait disorder with apraxic features. At times, the disability fluctuated. On examination, her Mini-Mental State Examination score (which examines orientation, memory, attention, recall and language) was 18 out of 30; any score below 23 suggests a disturbance of cognition. She had first-degree jerk nystagmus to the right, limb ataxia and extensor plantar responses. The patient's gait was apraxic, with a tendency to be rooted to the spot, unable to progress either forwards or backwards. Findings from CSF studies and MRI were typical of MS.

Mental impairment can begin early in the course of MS and does not correlate with the degree of physical disability.

abnormality may be unilateral or bilateral. Patients seldom complain of diplopia, but some notice problems with the tracking of moving objects (Figure 3.3).

Case history 3.2 – visual function

A 38-year-old man was diagnosed as having MS 14 years previously. He had no specific visual complaints. His arms felt strong, but he was aware of tingling and numbness in the fingertips. He was just able to stand with a frame, but found walking extremely difficult. His legs were liable to stiffen or jerk. The patient complained of urgency of micturition coupled with incontinence but, at other times, hesitancy. He had also been chronically constipated. He had experienced erectile dysfunction for some time. Examination showed bilateral optic disc pallor but no other cranial-nerve abnormality. His upper limbs were spastic and he had a mild pyramidal weakness coupled with cerebellar ataxia. He had impaired proprioception in the fingers, and a severe spastic paraparesis, with a markedly impaired sense of vibration throughout the legs, and a reduced sense of joint position in the feet.

Optic disc pallor is a highly subjective physical sign, but it is evident that all MS patients eventually have optic nerve pathology, whether or not they have had attacks of optic neuritis.

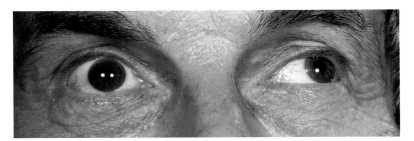

Figure 3.3 Internuclear ophthalmoplegia. On attempted lateral gaze the patient displays nystagmus in the left (abducting) eye and impaired adduction of the right eye.

Questions that patients often ask

Is the disease hereditary?
Genetic factors play a part in determining susceptibility to MS (see Table 1.1, page 9).

What is the effect of pregnancy?
Relapse frequency does not increase during pregnancy itself, but it does increase in the first 3 months of the puerperium. There are no data to suggest that MS has an adverse effect on the fetus, or that the long-term outcome of MS is influenced by previous obstetric history.

Can I have vaccinations?
There is no firm evidence that single vaccinations trigger an acute exacerbation of MS or alter its long-term outcome.

Can I have an anesthetic?
There is no evidence that either general or local anesthesia triggers exacerbations of the disease.

Should I avoid any dental procedures?
Dental procedures do not affect the course of the condition, and no special precautions are needed for most patients with MS. In addition, there is no evidence to justify the removal of intact mercury-containing amalgam fillings to improve MS.

Should I go on a diet?
There is little evidence to support any requirement for dietary change in patients with MS. However, many patients move to a diet low in animal fats, with supplements of polyunsaturated fatty acids (e.g. linoleic acid, linolenic acid and arachidonic acid).

Favored supplements include sunflower seed and evening primrose oils. The diets are, in a sense, healthy ones, but there are very few data to support their use. Maintaining an ideal bodyweight and good conditioning is important.

There is no evidence to support a switch to a gluten-free diet.

Should I have oxygen therapy?
Although an early study suggested that hyperbaric (high-pressure) oxygen therapy was beneficial, the findings could not be reproduced.

Can I drive?

Regulations vary from country to country. In both the UK and the USA, a driver may retain their license (which normally expires when the driver reaches the age of 70 years) after a medical assessment confirms that driving performance is not impaired. Under certain circumstances, specially adapted vehicles may be recommended. In the UK, if the diagnosis is recent or there is evidence of rapid disease progression, a short-period license (1, 2 or 3 years) will be issued. For heavy goods vehicles, a 1-year license may be issued subject to the condition being stable and there being no driving impairment.

It is not always possible to judge the influence of neurological disabilities on the ability to respond appropriately in real driving situations. For this reason, it is advisable to observe patients under simulated and actual road conditions to determine whether they can handle a vehicle safely.

Can trauma bring on new symptoms?

This remains a controversial issue and receives regular airing in courts of law. Some patients have described the development of a focal neurological deficit related to the site of recent trauma (Case history 3.3), but epidemiological data do not support a link between trauma and the precipitation or worsening of MS.

Case history 3.3 – effect of trauma

A 19-year-old woman received blows to the left shoulder and face while playing hockey. A few hours later she developed blurred vision in the left eye, associated with pain on eye movement. She had had an episode of optic neuritis in the right eye 2 years earlier. On examination, the right disc was pale and the left disc was slightly swollen. The patient had a left relative afferent pupillary defect and reduced visual acuity to the perception of hand movements only. The patient's vision failed to recover. On the basis of sequential attacks of optic neuritis, she was diagnosed as having MS.

Although acute attacks of MS can appear to be related in time to acute trauma, there is no convincing evidence of a correlation between the two.

Motor function

A small proportion of patients with longstanding MS may show either depressed reflexes or wasting. For most, however, the motor deficit is pyramidal, and characterized by a spastic paraparesis of varying degree. Typical findings include spastic legs, ankle clonus and bilateral extensor plantar responses. Over time, patients become increasingly reliant on either walking aids or the use of a wheelchair. Involvement of the upper limbs is more variable and, fortunately, seldom reaches a degree that renders the patient totally dependent.

Cerebellar function

Limb ataxia is commonplace in established MS. When it is severe, it interferes substantially with everyday function. Truncal ataxia may be disproportionate to limb involvement, so that the predominant disturbance is to the patient's gait. A cerebellar dysarthria is likely if the limb findings are prominent.

In addition to nystagmus, cerebellar ocular signs include broken pursuit movement and overshooting or undershooting saccades. Only rarely is the disability purely cerebellar in the later stages of the disease.

Sphincter function

Bladder symptoms are common in the established condition. Retention is unusual – most patients complain of a mixture of frequency and urgency, often coupled with hesitancy. This curious combination arises from a lack of coordination between bladder contraction and sphincter relaxation: the detrusor muscle contracts (triggering the urgency), but the sphincter fails to relax (triggering the hesitancy). Fecal urgency and incontinence are mercifully uncommon.

Sexual function

Erectile dysfunction has been reported in up to 40% of male patients, and correlates with the presence of sphincter impairment (see Sexual problems, page 59).

Key points – the established condition

- Intellectual changes may appear relatively early in the course of the disease and do not correlate with levels of physical disability.
- The influence of pregnancy on the disease and the risk of MS being inherited by offspring must be discussed with patients who are planning a family.
- Patients should be advised that vaccinations, dental procedures and anesthesia can be carried out without risk of affecting the disease.
- Dietary manipulation has, at most, a marginal effect on the course of the disease.

Key references

Confavreux C, Hutchinson M, Hours MM et al. Rate of pregnancy-related relapse in multiple sclerosis. N Engl J Med 1998;339:285–91.

Runmarker B, Andersen O. Prognostic factors in a multiple sclerosis incidence cohort with twenty-five years of follow-up. Brain 1993;116:117–34.

Sadovnick AD, Armstrong H, Rice GPA et al. A population-based study of multiple sclerosis in twins: update. Ann Neurol 1993;33: 281–5.

Sibley WA, Bamford CR, Clark K et al. A prospective study of physical trauma and multiple sclerosis. J Neurol Neurosurg Psychiatry 1991;54:584–9.

Vickrey BG, Hays RD, Harooni R et al. A health-related quality of life measure for multiple sclerosis. Qual Life Res 1995;4:187–206.

The diagnosis of multiple sclerosis (MS) rests on the principle that the clinician can demonstrate dissemination of the disease in both space and time. Clinically, this means that the patient has episodes (or attacks) of neurological dysfunction that occur:
- in different parts of the central nervous system (CNS) (dissemination in space)
- at intervals separated by at least a month of complete recovery, or intervals in which the dysfunction from a previous attack clearly stabilizes (dissemination in time).

This principle formed the basis of previous criteria proposed by Schumacher in 1965 and subsequently extended by Poser in 1983.

Paraclinical investigation by modern neuroimaging and the selected use of electrophysiological testing, together with careful laboratory analysis of cerebrospinal fluid (CSF), has greatly enhanced confidence in the diagnosis of MS. Furthermore, the results of magnetic resonance imaging (MRI) at first presentation have predictive value when the presenting symptoms are highly suggestive of an inflammatory demyelinating disease.

New diagnostic criteria were published in 2001 by the International Panel on the Diagnosis of Multiple Sclerosis, chaired by Professor WI McDonald of the Royal College of Physicians, London. Known as the London Panel or McDonald criteria, these guidelines formally incorporate MRI findings into the diagnostic algorithm and are now generally widely accepted.

The criteria are periodically revisited by the panel with the goal of further clarification. The criteria were most recently reviewed and revised in 2005 based on evidence from clinical investigations and experience gained since the introduction of the new guidelines in 2001. In the revision, the MRI criteria for dissemination in space better define the use of spinal imaging, while the MRI criteria for dissemination in time have been simplified. In addition, the CSF requirement for primary progressive MS has been relaxed.

Diagnostic criteria

The new London Panel criteria (Table 4.1) retain the useful features of previous criteria. They also:

- provide guidelines appropriate for practitioners, while allowing adaptability for research purposes
- clarify definitions used in diagnosis
- integrate the use of MRI (Table 4.2)
- incorporate criteria for primary progressive disease
- provide an evidence-based platform for diagnosis when possible
- take potential limits on diagnostic resources into account.

TABLE 4.1

London Panel (McDonald) criteria for diagnosis of MS

Attacks*	Lesions†	Additional requirement
≥ 2	≥ 2	None, after other conditions are excluded MRI and CSF are desirable, but not required
≥ 2	1	Dissemination in space documented by MRI, *or* positive CSF and ≥ 2 MRI lesions, *or* a subsequent clinical attack in a different site
1	≥ 2	Dissemination in time documented by MRI, *or* a subsequent clinical attack
1‡	1	Dissemination in space documented by MRI, *or* positive CSF and ≥ 2 MRI lesions, *and* dissemination in time documented by MRI, *or* a subsequent clinical attack
0§	1	At least 1 year of disease progression (recorded by history or observed) *and* two or three of the following: (i) ≥ 9 MRI lesions, *or* ≥ 4 MRI lesions and a positive VER (ii) ≥ 2 focal lesions on spinal MRI (iii) positive CSF

*An episode of objectively verified neurological dysfunction of the type typical of MS that lasts a minimum of 24 hours.
†Inferred by objective evidence of abnormalities found on neurological examination.
‡Clinically isolated syndrome of the type suggestive of MS.
§Progressive disease from onset; primary progressive or progressive relapsing MS.
CSF, cerebrospinal fluid; MRI, magnetic resonance imaging; VER, visual evoked response.

TABLE 4.2

London Panel dissemination criteria for MS from the findings of MRI

In space, any three of:

≥ 1 lesion on a gadolinium-enhanced T1-weighted MRI scan

≥ 9 lesions on a T2-weighted MRI scan

≥ 1 infratentorial lesion(s)

≥ 1 juxtacortical lesion(s)

≥ 3 periventricular lesions

In time, either of:

≥ 1 gadolinium-enhanced lesion on a T1-weighted MRI scan ≥ 3 months after a clinical attack

≥ 1 new lesion on a T2-weighted MRI scan performed at any time after a reference MRI scan obtained at least 30 days after a clinical attack

Note: A focal T2 lesion on a spinal MRI scan counts as an infratentorial lesion, contributes to the total number of lesions and, if enhancing, satisfies the gadolinium-enhanced lesion criteria.

The criteria retain dissemination in space and time as a required cornerstone of diagnosis, and demand that clinical evidence rests on demonstrated clinical signs and not historical accounts of symptoms. They also require exclusion of other explanations of each patient's clinical features and laboratory findings.

The levels of diagnostic certainty are now defined as:

- MS, which incorporates most of what was previously referred to as clinically definite, laboratory-supported definite or clinically probable MS in the Poser criteria
- possible MS, for the patient who is still under evaluation for MS but has not yet fulfilled the criteria
- not MS.

The utility of these new criteria is supported by retrospective analysis of prospectively acquired data on the natural history of cases at first presentation, and from analysis of longitudinal data from selected treatment trials.

Paraclinical criteria

Neurophysiological tests. Slowing of impulse transmission along rapidly conducting, myelinated, large-fiber pathways is a hallmark of demyelination. Conduction velocities over several CNS sensory pathways can be reproducibly measured using generally available techniques. The selected use of evoked potentials (visual, auditory and somatosensory) can confirm the diagnosis of MS. However, testing should not duplicate established clinical findings. For example, in a patient with optic neuritis, slowing of conduction on visual evoked responses does not imply an additional CNS lesion. In contrast, in a patient with a normal neurological examination result outside the visual system, abnormalities on somatosensory evoked responses provide paraclinical evidence of subclinical involvement of the spinal cord that increases diagnostic certainty.

Magnetic stimulation of the motor cortex is a potentially useful test for evaluating the integrity of conduction over central pyramidal pathways; however, the test is not broadly available.

Visual evoked potentials are generally the most reliable and cost-effective of these paraclinical tests.

Magnetic resonance imaging is the most useful investigative tool when MS is suspected. It has greatly advanced our understanding of the dynamics of lesion formation in the disease. Disease activity in relapsing forms of MS, as monitored by serial MRI, is five to ten times more frequent than is suggested by clinical attack rates. As a neuroimaging modality, MRI has great sensitivity for detecting the types of lesions seen in MS. Unfortunately, the abnormalities found on MRI scans – particularly those seen on a single examination – are not specific for the disease. Nonetheless, certain combinations of findings on cerebral MRI have high specificity for MS (Figure 4.1), although they are not often present early in the disease course.

Selective imaging of the spinal cord and optic nerves may be useful in some patients. Directed examination of these areas is more fruitful in individual cases, for example, when anatomic definition of lesions is required for differential diagnostic purposes. Imaging of the spinal cord may be particularly helpful when cerebral imaging

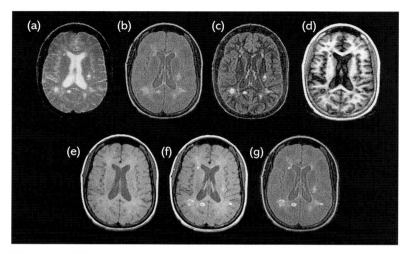

Figure 4.1 MRI scans from a 39-year-old woman with remitting relapsing MS and an Expanded Disability Status Score of 1.5. She had experienced increased fatigue, and new numbness and clumsiness of her right leg. MS was suspected when she experienced her first bout of sensory symptoms and mild sensory loss 11 years earlier. The MRI slices were taken using the following pulse sequences: (a) T2-weighted; (b) fluid attenuation by inversion recovery (FLAIR); (c) dual-inversion recovery for the suppression of normal white matter and CSF; (d) dual-inversion recovery for the suppression of gray matter and CSF; (e) unenhanced T1-weighted; (f) post gadolinium-enhanced T1-weighted; (g) a composite image of the map of the gadolinium-enhanced tissue (yellow) superimposed onto the FLAIR images of the lesions. Some of the MS plaques are enhanced, signifying inflammatory activity. Many have different appearances on images obtained by different sequences, regardless of their enhancement status. This variable pattern is characteristic of MS.

shows a pattern that might be more consistent with small-vessel disease. While spinal-cord lesions are uncommon in patients with vascular disease, they are frequently found in patients with MS.

In general, cerebral MRI alone is most cost-effective for routine initial diagnosis. However, lesions found on spinal MRI scans may help to fulfill new MRI criteria for dissemination in space, and can be especially valuable in older individuals, as non-specific intramedullary lesions are uncommon in the spinal cord.

Lesions are most often represented by high-signal-intensity ovoids in periventricular and subcortical white matter on T2-weighted images. After administration of paramagnetic contrast agents composed of irreversible chelates of gadolinium, active lesions are enhanced on T1-weighted images. Some lesions are seen as regions of reduced signal intensity on T1-weighted images. When these lesions persist over multiple examinations, they signify chronic plaques that pathologically show substantial tissue disruption and axonal loss; persistent 'black holes' correlate with greater clinical disability. Typical lesions in clinically definite MS found by MRI are shown in Figure 4.1.

Laboratory criteria

MS patients as a group have a number of immunologic and immunochemical abnormalities, none of which distinguishes individual patients from those with other neurological diseases or from healthy individuals. All CSF abnormalities are non-specific. However, in an appropriate clinical setting, some CSF parameters can increase the likelihood of diagnosis.

Cerebrospinal fluid. In MS, CSF often reveals a mild, mononuclear-cell pleocytosis, and total protein concentration is slightly elevated. However, it is unusual to find more than 50 cells/mm^3 or protein content above 100 mg/100 mL in MS, and such measurements should alert the clinician to a possible alternative diagnosis.

During processes that damage myelin, myelin basic protein and other myelin proteins are released into the CSF, where they can be measured. Intrathecal synthesis of immunoglobulin is always an abnormal finding. This is measurable with increasing sensitivity by determination of:

- CSF gamma globulins as a percentage of total protein
- an index of the amount of CSF immunoglobulin G (IgG) normalized to the amount of CSF and serum albumin and IgG
- the rate of synthesis of CSF IgG.

The IgG index and synthetic rates are highly reproducible in commercial laboratories. However, finding bands of limited heterogeneity (i.e. oligoclonal bands) is dependent on technique, and sensitivity varies with the experience and care of the reference laboratory. In research centers, oligoclonal bands are found in approximately 95% of patients with clinically definite MS.

At diagnosis, CSF evaluation is most helpful in those patients with only a single clinically defined objective lesion and few typical lesions identified by MRI. The CSF must be abnormal to permit a diagnosis of MS in patients who have progressive disease from the onset (see Table 4.1).

Clinical staging

A number of scales have been adopted in an attempt to stage the accumulation of neurological findings, disability and impairment in patients with MS. These have been developed primarily for use in clinical trials, and are not routinely used in clinical practice. All the scales have a number of notable limitations. Nevertheless, the Expanded Disability Status Score (EDSS) has been used so often that it has attained, by default, gold-standard status for judging the outcomes of clinical trials. To understand the results of clinical trials and to put individual patients into perspective regarding natural history studies, some working knowledge of the EDSS system is useful, even if it is not universally embraced in the day-to-day management of patients.

Expanded Disability Status Score. The EDSS is based on:
- a neurological examination
- a formalized assessment of symptoms
- an evaluation of the patient's global abilities (e.g. to walk or transfer independently, or with help).

Recent clinical studies have put additional restrictions and definitions on the original EDSS. These changes are designed to improve the reproducibility of the EDSS when applied by different investigators in multicenter trials. Some of these changes are subtle and others are more obvious, but all may lead to somewhat different behavior of the scoring system, which may account for variations in outcome between studies using similar therapeutic agents.

The classic EDSS is an amalgamation of scoring in eight predefined functional systems:
- pyramidal
- sensory
- cerebellar
- bowel and bladder
- brainstem
- visual
- mental
- other.

This last category of 'other' functions is poorly defined. Scoring of the functional systems ranges from normal (0) to severe disability (5 or 6 depending on the system). The EDSS ranges from 0 (a normal neurological examination result and no bowel or bladder symptoms) to 10 (death due to MS), with 18 intermediate steps at 0.5-unit increments from 1.0 (Table 4.3).

TABLE 4.3

Definition of Expanded Disability Status Score (EDSS)

EDSS	Extent of disability
0–1.5	Neurological findings without associated disability
2.0–3.0	Neurological findings with patient aware of some mild disability
3.5 and 4.0	Increasing disability in one or more functional systems; in general, the patient has an unrestricted gait and good endurance
4.5	Limitations in distance walked begin to affect scoring
5.0 and 5.5	Increasing disabilities in one or more functional systems; relates to distance that can be walked without resting
6.0 and 6.5	Unilateral or bilateral assistance needed for ambulation, respectively
7.0 and 7.5	Wheelchair needed, with or without transfer assistance
8.0 and above	Increasingly severe bed- or chairbound status, with increasing dependence on others for all functions

The EDSS is associated with a number of difficulties. Although the scoring system reflects a continuum of accumulated disability (ordinal data), the steps in the EDSS scale are not necessarily equal (continuous data). This leads to problems in the statistical analysis of group data based on the EDSS. It also leads to some aberrations in the scores assigned to some patients. In addition, by using the EDSS to select patients for clinical trials, a patient's entry to a trial can be restricted depending on their ability to walk without assistive devices (level 5.5) or on any limitations of endurance (level 5.0), or on their ability to walk at least 5 m (16.5 ft) even if bilateral assistance is required (level 6.5). The same criteria have subsequently been artificially imposed by regulatory agencies and third-party payers for limiting the use of newer immunomodulatory drugs to certain subgroups of patients with MS.

Prognosis at presentation

Individuals often present with clinical syndromes that are highly suggestive of MS, but a clinically definite diagnosis cannot be established (see Table 4.1). These patients include those with monosymptomatic presentations, such as optic neuritis, syndromes involving an incomplete spinal cord (e.g. partial transverse myelitis) and certain brainstem syndromes (internuclear ophthalmoplegia, facial myokymia and isolated limb ataxia). In these individuals, the MRI findings at presentation are useful in assessing the risk of developing a disease-defining clinical or subclinical MRI event, and for the risk of developing fixed neurological disability over the next 2–14 years.

The presence and number of lesions on cerebral MRI scans are useful in predicting moderate to high risk. The absence of abnormalities on a cerebral MRI scan suggests a low risk of progression to clinically definite disease or modest disability.

In patients with optic neuritis and no abnormalities on cerebral MRI scans, the presence or absence of oligoclonal bands in the CSF refines the risk levels for the next few years. There are no available data to suggest that MRI findings are useful prognostic indicators of future disease course for individual patients with well-established MS.

Key points – diagnosis

- The diagnostic criteria for MS have been revised to include the use of magnetic resonance imaging (MRI) in documenting disease dissemination in space and time, generally facilitating more rapid diagnosis.
- Subclinical disease activity on MRI greatly exceeds clinical activity.
- A diagnosis of MS in the absence of typical MRI findings or cerebrospinal fluid analysis should be treated with suspicion.
- The diagnosis of MS can never be based solely on MRI findings.
- The number and volume of lesions on cerebral MRI scans at initial clinical presentation is highly predictive of the short-term, but not the longer-term, course of the disease.

Key references

Bot JC, Barkhof F, Polman CH et al. Spinal cord abnormalities in recently diagnosed MS patients: added value of spinal MRI examination. *Neurology* 2004;62:226–33.

Brex PA, Ciccarelli O, O'Riordan JI et al. A longitudinal study of abnormalities on MRI and disability from multiple sclerosis. *N Engl J Med* 2002;346:158–64.

Dalton CM, Brex PA, Miszkiel KA et al. Application of the new McDonald criteria to patients with clinically isolated syndromes suggestive of multiple sclerosis. *Ann Neurol* 2002;52:47–53.

Gronseth GS, Ashman EJ. Practice parameter: the usefulness of evoked potentials in identifying clinically silent lesions in patients with suspected multiple sclerosis (an evidence-based review): report of the Quality Standards Subcommittee of the American Academy of Neurology. *Neurology* 2000;54:1720–5.

Jin YP, de Pedro-Cuesta J, Huang YH, Soderstrom M. Predicting multiple sclerosis at optic neuritis onset. *Mult Scler* 2003;9:135–41.

Kurtzke JF. The Disability Status Scale for multiple sclerosis: apologia pro DSS sua. *Neurology* 1989;39:291–302.

McDonald WI, Compston A, Edan G et al. Recommended diagnostic criteria for multiple sclerosis: guidelines from the International Panel on the Diagnosis of Multiple Sclerosis. *Ann Neurol* 2001;50: 121–7.

Polman CH, Reingold SC, Edan G et al. Diagnostic criteria for multiple sclerosis: 2005 revisions to the "McDonald criteria". *Ann Neurol* 2005 (In press). Available online at www3.interscience.wiley.com/cgi-bin/jissue/78504407

Polman CH, Reingold SC, Wolinsky JS. MS diagnostic criteria: three years later. *Multipl Scler* 2005;11:5–12.

Tintore M, Rovira A, Rio J et al. New diagnostic criteria for multiple sclerosis: application in first demyelinating episode. *Neurology* 2003;60:27–30.

Wolinsky JS; PROMiSe Study Group. The diagnosis of primary progressive multiple sclerosis. *J Neurol Sci* 2003;206:145–52.

Acute attacks

Of the potential treatments, corticosteroid therapy has
demonstrated the most convincing effect on both the severity and
the duration of acute attacks. Controversy remains regarding the
most effective type of steroid, and whether the type of steroid used
has any influence on the subsequent disease course.

Choice of treatment. The first properly randomized double-blind
study of steroids for acute exacerbations of multiple sclerosis (MS)
used corticotropin (adrenocorticotropic hormone) over a 2-week
period. Treated patients showed some advantage over untreated
patients in the first 2 weeks, predominantly in terms of motor,
sensory and sphincter function. Although the analysis ceased 4 weeks
after entry to the trial, the data suggested that there would have been
no significant difference between the treated and untreated groups
soon afterwards. Subsequently, oral steroids were used on the
assumption that an oral preparation was as effective as corticotropin.

Controlled studies later concluded that intravenous
methylprednisolone, 500–1000 mg daily for 3–7 days, was
superior to placebo, but not necessarily superior to corticotropin.
Compared with either oral prednisolone or placebo, intravenous
methylprednisolone has been found to hasten return of normal
vision in patients with optic neuritis, but to have no influence
on the long-term outcome in terms of residual visual deficits. A
further study failed to demonstrate an advantage of intravenous
methylprednisolone over the oral formulation in patients with MS,
although the subjects in this study may have been treated rather
late after the onset of symptoms.

A complicating factor when deciding which steroid preparation
to use is that, for some types of attack, the mode of treatment
influences the subsequent course of the disease. In one study in
which patients with optic neuritis were treated with placebo, oral

steroids or intravenous steroids, twice as many patients treated with the placebo or oral steroid developed MS over a 2-year follow-up period than in the group that received intravenous steroid at the time of the acute attack. By 4 years' follow-up, however, the rate of MS development was similar in all three treatment groups.

There is no consensus as to which regimen should be used. For severely disabling attacks, most neurologists use intravenous methylprednisolone, 500–1000 mg daily for 3–5 days. For less disabling attacks for which treatment is still considered justified, oral prednisolone, 60 mg daily, can be used for a week, followed by 30 mg daily for another week and 15 mg daily for a final week.

Patient selection. Which patients with acute attacks should be treated? In general, it seems reasonable to confine treatment to those patients whose attacks are disabling but who do not necessarily require admission to hospital. If, on the other hand, the attack has not had a significant effect on lifestyle, steroid therapy hardly seems worthwhile.

Treatment of symptoms

Fatigue is a common complaint in patients with MS. Studies have suggested that amantadine, 100 mg twice daily, and possibly the central nervous system (CNS) stimulant modafinil, 200 mg daily, can lessen this symptom. In a double-blind study, neither of these drugs was found to affect attention, visual or verbal memory, or motor speed. Any effect after treatment with amantadine is usually evident within a month.

Motor, visual or cerebellar function. Aminopyridines (potassium-channel blockers) enhance nerve conduction in the CNS. 4-Aminopyridine in a dose of up to 0.5 mg/kg/day has been shown to have some objective effect on extraocular motility, strength, coordination, gait and visual function in patients with MS. The effects are small and the drug is not used routinely. It is not licensed in the UK or USA.

Spasticity. The main drugs used for the treatment of spasticity are shown in Table 5.1. They are:

- diazepam
- baclofen
- dantrolene sodium
- tizanidine.

Occasionally, with any of these drugs, patients can experience striking flaccidity, a disadvantage if weakness is also a problem.

Oral agents. Baclofen is probably the drug of choice, starting at a dose of around 15 mg daily; the dose should be increased slowly, otherwise sedation becomes a major problem (Case history 5.1).

TABLE 5.1

Antispasticity agents

Diazepam	Baclofen	Dantrolene sodium	Tizanidine
Daily dose			
2–15 mg, divided doses	15–100 mg, divided doses	25–400 mg, divided doses	2–36 mg, divided doses
Mode of action			
Acts on GABA-mediated inhibitory circuits	Acts as a GABA agonist at a spinal level	Acts peripherally on inhibitory circuits	α2-adreno-receptor agonist at a spinal level
Common side effects			
Drowsiness	Sedation	Drowsiness	Dry mouth
Confusion	Drowsiness	Dizziness	Somnolence
Ataxia	Nausea	Fatigue	Asthenia
Paradoxical increase in aggression	Lassitude	Diarrhea	Dizziness
Dependency	Dizziness	Nausea	Headache
	Ataxia	Headache	
	Depression	Liver dysfunction	
	Tremor		

GABA, gamma-aminobutyric acid.

Rapid withdrawal of the drug can lead to a rebound increase in spasticity. Diazepam is an alternative agent, but high doses are often required. Clonazepam is sometimes used. Dantrolene acts peripherally. Tizanidine, which is related to clonidine, has a notable effect on spasticity.

Intrathecal agents. If oral preparations are unhelpful, and the spasticity is disabling, intrathecal baclofen can be considered. This technique substantially relieves spasticity, as well as spontaneous spasms and pain. Complications of the technique include wound infection, pump malfunctions and low-pressure headache due to cerebrospinal fluid leakage.

Intravenous agents. Botulinum toxin type A is, at least theoretically, a potential treatment for spasticity. Objective improvement in spasticity is demonstrable, but considerable quantities of the drug are required for treatment of the leg muscles, and injections are needed every 3 months or so.

Case history 5.1 – spasticity

A 52-year-old woman had had MS for 15 years. She had entered the secondary progressive phase of the disease, and her walking distance was limited to about 100 m using a walking aid. She was troubled by leg stiffness and also experienced painful flexor spasms of the legs at night. She was started on baclofen 5 years earlier and had been taking 30 mg daily for 3 years with no clear benefit.

After a review of the patient's progress with a neurologist, the dose of baclofen was gradually increased to see if a higher intake might provide some benefit. After some troublesome side effects (drowsiness and nausea) while the dose was raised, the patient was able to tolerate 80 mg daily; at that dose she found her flexor spasms had virtually disappeared.

Antispastic agents are often of very limited benefit in patients with MS, but before abandoning their use the clinician should pursue a particular drug regimen to the limits of the patient's tolerance.

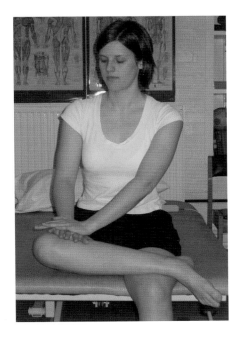

Figure 5.1 Piriformis and partial adductor stretch for the relief of spasticity.

Non-pharmacological treatment. The role of physiotherapy, with or without an antispastic agent, has been appraised. Evidence suggests that the beneficial effects of baclofen on spasticity can be enhanced by the concomitant use of stretching exercises (Figure 5.1).

Bladder symptoms are very common in established MS. The most characteristic complaint is of urgency and frequency, sometimes combined with incontinence, but on other occasions with hesitancy and a poor stream. The symptoms are often the result of a lack of coordination between detrusor contraction and bladder-neck relaxation.

Before embarking on drug therapy, an understanding of the type of bladder disorder is essential. Appraisal of symptoms alone is not enough, and clinicians should always investigate bladder status. Ultrasound analysis of bladder volume both before and after micturition is invaluable (Figure 5.2), and may suffice for rational management. However, sometimes cystometry is also required. The discovery of a large residual volume after micturition is a relative contraindication to the use of certain drugs. Available drugs act at different sites of the neurogenic pathway that controls micturition (Table 5.2; Figure 5.3).

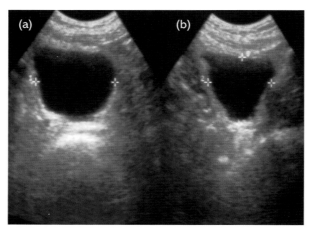

Figure 5.2 Ultrasound scans showing the bladder (a) before micturition and (b) after micturition, with a large residual volume. The cursors (+) mark the bladder-wall boundaries.

TABLE 5.2

Drugs for bladder symptoms

Drug	Site and mode of action
Anticholinergics (e.g. propantheline, oxybutynin, tolterodine)	Reduce detrusor hyperreflexia
Cholinergics	Enhance detrusor activity
α-sympathetic blockers (e.g. indoramin)	Relax smooth muscle, including the internal sphincter
Antispastic agents (e.g. baclofen)	Relax tone in the external sphincter
Vasopressin analogs (e.g. desmopressin)	Reduce urine production (for the management of nocturia)

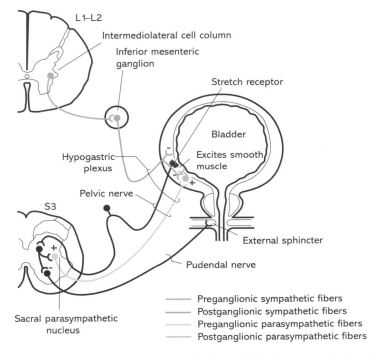

Figure 5.3 Bladder innervation: parasympathetic stimulation leads to contraction of the smooth muscle and relaxation of the urethra, resulting in voiding, while the role of sympathetic innervation of the bladder neck in preserving continence remains uncertain.

Urge incontinence. For patients with urge incontinence (due to detrusor hyperreflexia), the drugs of choice are:
- oxybutynin, 5–15 mg daily (in divided doses)
- propantheline, 30–90 mg daily (in divided doses)
- tolterodine, 2–4 mg daily (in divided doses).

Alternatively, a tricyclic antidepressant (e.g. amitriptyline) may be given as a single dose at night. The use of all of these drugs is limited by anticholinergic side effects (e.g. dry mouth and constipation). If they lead to an increasing urinary residual volume, their use must be reconsidered (Case history 5.2). Desmopressin, 10–20 µg at night, is helpful in younger patients with nocturnal frequency and incontinence. Care should be taken to avoid fluid overload.

> **Case history 5.2 – bladder dysfunction**
>
> A 40-year-old woman had had MS for 6 years; bladder symptoms
> had become prominent over the previous 12 months. She
> complained to her primary care provider of marked urgency and
> frequency, but felt that she was emptying her bladder completely.
> Oxybutynin, 2.5 mg three times daily, was administered to see if
> the drug would provide any benefit. A week later, the patient
> developed urinary retention and had to present at her local
> hospital for catheterization.
>
> *Symptoms are an inadequate guide to the pathophysiology of*
> *bladder disturbance. Ultrasound should be undertaken before and*
> *after micturition, before treatment is initiated.*

Incomplete emptying. These patients (e.g. with residual volume
exceeding 100 mL), probably need intermittent catheterization.
However, before taking this course of action, the patient can try
to encourage bladder emptying by stimulating the anal region
or the lower abdomen. If this fails, it is worth considering a trial
of an α-adrenergic blocking agent, such as indoramin, 20–100 mg
daily.

Intermittent self-catheterization becomes necessary if there is a
persistent and significant residual volume after micturition. As long
as the patient has reasonable vision and hand control, the procedure
can be readily learned, and the incidence of bladder infection is far
lower than with indwelling or suprapubic catheters. The patient
should be advised to maintain a high fluid intake.

Urinary tract infections. Despite the above precautions, urinary
tract infections still occur. Urine culture is essential before starting
therapy. Many infections respond to ampicillin, nalidixic acid,
nitrofurantoin or trimethoprim, for 1 week, but resistant organisms
are common. If the patient develops frequent, symptomatic
infections, consider long-term, low-dose antibiotic therapy
(e.g. trimethoprim or nitrofurantoin, 50–100 mg at night).

Surgery. When all other measures have failed, various forms of surgical intervention may be used. In one procedure, bladder-neck closure is accompanied by the introduction of a suprapubic catheter. Neural prostheses have been used in an attempt to stimulate bladder voiding, but have been mainly used in patients with spinal-cord trauma.

Bowel problems. Fecal incontinence is relatively uncommon. When present, it usually accompanies urinary urgency and incontinence. Constipation is a more common problem, often compounded by the anticholinergic properties of some of the drugs used for symptom control. Most patients respond to an increase in dietary fiber or to osmotic laxatives such as lactulose or macrogols (inert polymers of ethylene glycol). Macrogols are administered with fluid and do not absorb further fluid from the body into the bowel.

Sexual problems. Some of the problems that MS patients experience with sexual intercourse relate either to loss of vaginal or penile sensation, or to the difficulties that spasticity imposes on the physical act itself. Erectile dysfunction can also be a problem. In the past, the most successful treatment has involved intracavernous injection of vasoactive drugs, such as papaverine. Hazards of the procedure include hematoma formation, local scarring and the induction of prolonged erections.

The phosphodiesterase type 5 inhibitors sildenafil, 50 mg, vardenafil, 10 mg, and tadalafil, 10 mg, are licensed for erectile dysfunction. They appear to be effective in at least some MS patients. Caution is necessary when using these drugs if the patient has concomitant cardiovascular disease.

Depression is more common than euphoria in patients with MS, and is more common in MS patients than in individuals with other neurological disorders that produce a comparable degree of disability (Case history 5.3). Its genesis, other than the immediate conclusion that it is triggered by a reaction to the illness itself, remains unknown.

Evidence to suggest that bipolar disorder is more common in patients with MS than in the general population is not persuasive.

Management is the same as for depression that occurs under other circumstances, although large doses of tricyclic anti-depressants may well produce troublesome side effects including sedation, dryness of the mouth, constipation and urinary retention.

Some patients exhibit pathological laughter and crying, which may respond to lower doses of amitriptyline.

Tremor. A severe, upper-limb tremor, particularly of the dominant hand, can lead to substantial disability. Drug therapy, for example with propranolol, is of only limited value. Thalamotomy (destruction of part of the thalamus) and thalamic pacing with implanted electrodes remain useful procedures in the management of this problem (Figure 5.4). Stereotactic lesions in the thalamus can have a dramatic effect on tremor without contributing to other disabilities of the limb.

Case history 5.3 – depression

A 50-year-old man had had MS for 18 years, and had substantial disability. On a routine visit to the neurology clinic, he was asked various questions about his situation and his capacity to cope with everyday activities. He indicated that his wife had left him months previously because of his problems, and that this, coupled with his disabilities, had had an adverse effect on his mood. He began to weep.

He was reassured and told that depression was an unusual feature in MS patients. He was advised to visit his primary care provider to discuss the matter further. A week later, the patient took an overdose of paracetamol, but recovered.

Depression is common in patients with MS, but is overlooked because it is not considered a common feature of the disease.

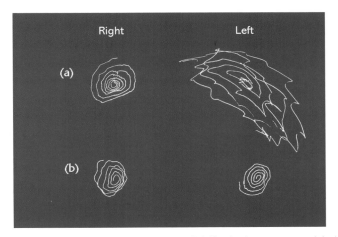

Figure 5.4 Spirals sketched by a patient with MS who has a tremor: (a) drawn before and (b) drawn after right thalamotomy.

Pain. Up to two-thirds of patients with MS experience pain at some stage of their illness; up to half of them complain of chronic pain. The pain may be paroxysmal or more persistent. The commonest paroxysmal pain is trigeminal neuralgia. Carbamazepine is the drug of choice, although its use may be limited by side effects including sedation and ataxia. Misoprostol, a long-acting synthetic prostaglandin E1 analog, 800 μg daily, has been shown to be effective.

The commonest chronic pain is one of burning sensations in the lower limbs, for which amitriptyline, up to 75 mg daily, is the drug of choice. Gabapentin, at an initial dose of 900 mg daily, may also be helpful in this setting.

Paroxysmal symptoms. Besides trigeminal neuralgia, other paroxysmal symptoms include painful tonic seizures, dysarthria and itching. These paroxysmal symptoms are usually abolished by low doses of carbamazepine (200–600 mg daily). Intravenous lidocaine or oral mexiletine, 300–400 mg daily, have similar effects. Intravenous lidocaine also appears to be effective in diminishing chronic positive symptoms, but mexiletine is less effective in this respect.

The role of cannabinoids

A recent study has been published on the effect of two different forms of cannabis on spasticity in patients with MS. There was no objective evidence of benefit, but some evidence of an improvement in terms of the patients' perception of the effects on spasticity, although it should be noted that it can often be difficult to mask from the patient whether they are receiving a cannabis derivative or a placebo. There was, however, some evidence of a small improvement in walking time in patients receiving active medication and also some benefit in terms of pain levels. This study seems to support some data from previous smaller studies, but there is still substantial uncertainty as to whether cannabis or its derivatives offer any meaningful benefit to patients with MS that could not be achieved by other means.

Key points – treatment of acute attacks and symptoms

- Corticosteroids shorten the duration of acute exacerbations of MS, but have no effect on the final outcome.
- Antispastic agents have only a limited role in the treatment of ambulant patients with MS.
- Intermittent self-catheterization is of great value for the control of bladder dysfunction in some patients with MS.
- Drugs that can play a role in the management of pain in MS include amitriptyline, carbamazepine and gabapentin.

Key references

Barnes D, Hughes RA, Morris RW et al. Randomised trial of oral and intravenous methylprednisolone in acute relapses of multiple sclerosis. *Lancet* 1997;349:902–6.

Fowler CJ. Neurological disorders of micturition and their treatment. *Brain* 1999;122:1213–31.

Moulin DE, Foley KM, Ebers GC. Pain syndromes in multiple sclerosis. *Neurology* 1988;38:1830–4.

Sadovnick AD, Remick RA, Allen J et al. Depression and multiple sclerosis. *Neurology* 1996;46: 628–32.

Thompson AJ. Multiple sclerosis: symptomatic treatment. *J Neurol* 1996;243:559–65.

Wasielewski PG, Burns JM, Koller WC. Pharmacologic treatment of tremor. *Mov Disord* 1998; 13 (suppl 3):90–100.

Zajicek J, Fox P, Sanders H et al. Cannabinoids for treatment of spasticity and other symptoms related to multiple sclerosis (CAMS study): multicentre randomised placebo-controlled trial. *Lancet* 2003;362:1517–26.

Until recently, there were no approved drugs to reduce the frequency of future multiple sclerosis (MS) attacks or the probability of accumulating neurological disability over time. Two classes of immunomodulatory drugs are now generally available:
• type I interferons (IFNs)
• glatiramer acetate (GA; copolymer-1).
A third drug, natalizumab, recently received accelerated approval in the USA, but was withdrawn from the market pending investigation of the emergence of progressive multifocal leukoencephalopathy (PML), an apparent complication of the therapy.

All drug classes reduce the risk of future attacks, and may also slow the rate of acquisition of neurological deficits.

Interferons

IFNs are produced naturally by the body. They were first recognized for their role in limiting certain viral infections. IFNs also alter the expression of surface molecules on, and the range of substances secreted by, immune cells. Many of these immunobiological effects, while not specific to particular antigens, are potentially relevant to MS.

A number of placebo-controlled clinical trials have been performed to investigate different recombinant IFN molecules. In general, type I IFNs (IFNα and IFNβ) reduce the frequency of clinical relapse, while type II IFNs (IFNγ) provoke attacks. The larger, published, pivotal trials have been limited to several forms of recombinant IFNβ. All of the trials were conducted in ambulatory patients with remitting relapsing disease and varying amounts of clinical disability. Several trials have also been completed on ambulatory patients with secondary progressive MS.

Benefits. There are three approved forms of recombinant IFNβ, which have somewhat different indications in different countries.

The approved formulations, standard dosage and current indications for use are provided in Table 6.1.

Effect on disease activity. Data from all controlled clinical trials in patients with relapsing forms of MS (encompassing clinically isolated syndromes with magnetic resonance imaging [MRI] evidence of risk of conversion to MS, relapsing remitting MS and secondary progressive MS with ongoing clinical relapses) support the use of IFNs to reduce clinical attack rates by about 30%. The trials also show that these drugs reduce the frequency of subclinical disease activity, as monitored by gadolinium enhancement and/or the appearance of new T2 lesions on MRI scans. The magnitudes of both the clinical and MRI-measured benefits seem to be both dose and frequency dependent. Higher doses of the same formulation produce larger effects; this effect is also seen when formulations of differing dose equivalents are compared. Although the best protection seems to be afforded by higher-dose and more frequently administered formulations, even lower-dose preparations reduce clinical relapses and the amount of MRI-monitored disease activity.

The effect of IFNβ treatment on clinical attacks and its MRI-measured benefits are attenuated for patients who develop sustained high titers of neutralizing antibodies; these antibodies are believed to be cross-reactive with the IFNβ formulations. Open-label extensions of the placebo-controlled pivotal trials suggest that the effects of treatment are sustained beyond the duration of the studies.

Effect on disability. Results from controlled trials indicate that the effect of IFNβ therapy on preventing the accumulation of disability or clinical disease progression is variable. Approximately 40% of all clinical relapses are associated with measurable neurological disability that persists for at least 3 months. Thus, the reduction of clinical attacks in patients with relapsing disease is likely to be associated with some attenuation of accumulated disability over time.

More contentious is whether the progression of disability that patients experience in the absence of well-defined clinical relapses can be treated with any of the IFNβ formulations. Studies in

TABLE 6.1

Available immunomodulators and indications in the UK and USA

Generic name	Proprietary name	Standard dosage	Indications*
Type I interferons			
IFNβ-1b	Betaferon (UK) Betaseron (USA)	250 μg s.c. on alternate days	Relapsing forms of MS to reduce the frequency of clinical exacerbations
IFNβ-1a	Rebif	44 μg s.c. 3 x weekly	Relapsing forms of MS to decrease the frequency of clinical exacerbations and delay the accumulation of physical disability; efficacy in chronic progressive MS has not been established
IFNβ-1a	Avonex	30 μg i.m. weekly	Relapsing forms of MS to slow the accumulation of physical disability and decrease the frequency of clinical exacerbations; efficacy has been demonstrated to include patients who have experienced a first clinical episode and have MRI features consistent with MS; safety and efficacy in patients with chronic progressive MS have not been established
Glatiramer			
Glatiramer acetate	Copaxone	20 mg s.c. daily	For reduction of the frequency of relapses in patients with remitting relapsing MS

TABLE 6.1 (CONTINUED)

Generic name	Proprietary name	Standard dosage	Indications*
Anti-α4-integrin humanized monoclonal antibody			
Natalizumab	Tysabri	300 mg i.v. every 4 weeks	For reduction of the frequency of relapses in patients with remitting relapsing MS

*General indication for both UK and USA (natalizumab is USA only, but current marketing is suspended); see individual product labeling for exact indication in country of use. IFN, interferon; i.m., intramuscular; i.v., intravenous; MRI, magnetic resonance imaging; s.c., subcutaneous.

patients with secondary progressive MS have shown trends for limited progression of disability, defined by the time to the appearance of an increase in neurological findings, as measured by a composite scale that is heavily weighted to impaired ambulation sustained over a 6-month interval. However, only one of these studies has reached statistical significance, and another was stopped prematurely on the basis of a futility analysis. Moreover, chronic measures of MRI-defined disease, including the progression of cerebral atrophy over time, have not supported a major drug effect on what are considered to be the most destructive aspects of MS. In conclusion, while the benefits of the IFNβ formulations on early relapsing remitting MS are well defined, they are less apparent in patients with disease that has entered a more progressive phase with infrequent continued clinical relapses. There are no data to support the use of IFNβ in patients with primary progressive MS.

Side effects of the three IFNβ preparations vary according to dose and route of administration. All of the preparations are associated with influenza-like side effects (including fever, malaise, and joint and muscle pain), which appear to be dose dependent.

The first injections may result in a transient worsening of neurological function that is probably related to the Uhthoff effect (a temporary deterioration of current, or reappearance of previous, neurological deficits in association with elevated body temperature). The intensity of these reactions usually weakens rapidly with subsequent injections.

Reactions at the injection site are common when IFNs are administered subcutaneously. They range from local redness at the injection site, with or without itching, to local induration of variable duration and severity, to local skin necrosis (Figure 6.1). The last is uncommon and is sometimes the consequence of unintended intracutaneous injections. Skin reactions and influenza-like symptoms usually decrease over time, but remain major causes of patient non-compliance during early treatment. Close patient contact and aggressive management of side effects during initiation of therapy may improve patient compliance.

Lymphopenia and elevations in hepatic enzyme levels are also dose-dependent side effects of therapy. These biochemical abnormalities seldom necessitate discontinuation of IFN treatment.

Less common side effects that arise later in therapy are exacerbation or unmasking of psoriasis and development of hypothyroidism. Preclinical studies in animals suggest that IFNβ may be an abortifacient; it is a category C drug for use in pregnancy.

Glatiramer acetate

GA (copolymer-1) binds strongly to molecules on the surfaces of antigen-presenting cells, which are central to the induction of a shift in naturally occurring GA-reactive T cells from a T helper type 1 (Th1) to a T helper type 2 (Th2) phenotype. These GA-reactive Th2 cells act to suppress myelin-antigen-reactive Th1 cells both systemically and within MS lesions. In animals, GA prevents immune-mediated neurological disease through the induction of organ-specific immunoregulatory GA-reactive Th2 cells. On passive transfer, these cells also exert neuroprotective effects through their secreted products in a number of models of retinal and central nervous system neural injury. Similar mechanisms may account for its effects in MS.

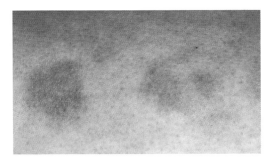

Figure 6.1 Skin reaction to subcutaneous injection of interferon.

Benefits. GA is indicated for the reduction of relapses in relapsing remitting MS. Treatment with GA reduces the number of clinical attacks and may slow accumulating clinical disability in ambulatory relapsing patients with mild-to-moderate clinical disability. Long-term follow-up studies support a persistent benefit over more than a decade of use. Several independent studies have shown that the clinical efficacy of GA is similar to that of the recombinant IFNβs (see Table 6.1). The effects of GA on MRI-monitored disease parameters parallel the clinical results. The drug reduces the numbers of enhanced lesions, T2 lesions and persisting new T1-hypointense lesions or 'black holes' (areas of potentially irreversible axon loss), and attenuates the development of cerebral atrophy. However, GA's role in the management of the progressive phase of MS is uncertain.

Side effects. There are few side effects associated with GA. Transient pain and/or minor swelling at the injection sites are common at the onset of therapy, but these diminish rapidly with time (Figure 6.2). Skin necrosis is not encountered.

Figure 6.2 Reaction to glatiramer therapy at injection site.

Neither influenza-like side effects nor abnormal laboratory results occur. However, 10–15% of patients treated with GA will eventually experience at least one systemic postinjection reaction, an injection response for which the mechanism of induction is not fully understood. During these reactions, patients report varied combinations of flushing, sweating, palpitations, a feeling of chest tightness and associated anxiety. The symptom complex usually resolves in a few minutes, but occasionally lasts several hours. These reactions are temporally associated with injection of the drug, are not seen with the first injection and do not occur on successive injections. They appear to be benign. Preclinical studies in animals suggest that GA is neither toxic nor teratogenic; it is a category B drug for use in pregnancy.

Natalizumab

Natalizumab is a recombinant humanized immunoglobulin G4κ monoclonal antibody that binds to the α4-subunit of α4β1 and α4β7 integrins, which are expressed on the surfaces of all leukocytes except neutrophils. Once bound, natalizumab inhibits the α4-mediated adhesion of leukocytes to their ligands. Most pertinent to MS, the adhesion of activated T cells to vascular endothelium via α4-integrin-mediated binding to vascular adhesion molecule-1 is impaired, thus preventing the transmigration of these cells across inflamed vessels into the brain. In vitro, natalizumab is known to bind to other molecules, including osteopontin; this binding may also play a role in the pathogenesis of MS.

Benefits. In late 2004, natalizumab received accelerated approval for use in the reduction of relapses in relapsing remitting MS in the USA. Approval by the Food and Drug Administration (FDA) was based on 1 year of data from two separate studies. The first compared natalizumab with placebo in patients with relapsing MS who were receiving no other therapy. The second compared natalizumab with placebo in MS patients who were receiving, and continued to be concomitantly treated with, IFNβ–1a (Avonex). Both studies showed a substantial reduction in annualized relapse rate at 1 year in natalizumab-treated patients compared with those receiving placebo or the active comparator by 66% and 54%, respectively. Acute measures of MRI activity were also attenuated for those patients receiving natalizumab. Both trials were continued in blinded fashion to determine if an effect on accumulating disability could also be demonstrated. Preliminary reports of 2-year data from these studies show that the effect on relapses and MRI metrics were maintained, and that accumulated disability was reduced by therapy. The role of natalizumab in the management of the progressive phase of MS is unknown.

Side effects. The primary conventional concern for therapy with natalizumab is the occurrence of allergic and hypersensitivity reactions (up to 7% of all subjects), including serious anaphylaxis/anaphylactoid reaction (0.8%). These reactions usually occur within 2 hours of the start of intravenous infusions of the drug and appear to be more common in patients who develop antibodies to the drug. Patients who experience these reactions are not to continue treatment with the drug.

Other side effects are few and minor, although an increased rate of infections may occur with this therapy. Preclinical studies in animals show that the drug undergoes transplacental transfer, exerting a number of reversible hematopoietic effects on the fetus. The drug is likely to be excreted in human milk. It is a category C drug for use in pregnancy.

Key points – treatment with immunomodulators

- Glatiramer acetate, all three formulations of recombinant interferon beta and natalizumab reduce the frequency of clinical attacks in relapsing MS.
- Approved immunomodulators are all injectables with acceptable side-effect profiles and good patient compliance.
- The benefit of the immunomodulators in progressive disease is limited.

In an extension study, PML, a generally rapidly progressive and fatal viral disease of the brain, developed in two MS subjects with more than 2 years' exposure to the combination of natalizumab and Avonex. PML was also reported in one subject with Crohn's disease who had received natalizumab with prior exposure to immunosuppressants.

At the time of publication (November 2005), marketing of the drug in the USA has been suspended pending a better understanding of the incidence of this complication. Researchers must determine whether risk management strategies might be adapted. Regardless of whether natalizumab can be reintroduced into the therapeutic armamentarium, the clinical results of these studies are harbingers of future generations of more effective therapeutic agents for MS.

Chemotherapeutic immunosuppressants

A broad variety of chemotherapeutic agents have been used in different strategies to attempt to control the disease. They range from relatively mild antimetabolites, such as azathioprine and methotrexate, to immunoablation with bone-marrow reconstitution. All are designed to attempt to re-establish a more normally responsive systemic immune system.

A full discussion of this treatment approach is beyond the scope of this chapter; however, one form of immunosuppressive chemotherapy, mitoxantrone, has received FDA approval in the USA for the indication of aggressive forms of relapsing MS based on a single phase III and supportive phase II study. The decision to advance to such aggressive therapy should be left to a specialist in the management of MS.

Key references

Cohen JA, Cutter GR, Fischer JS et al.; IMPACT Investigators. Benefit of interferon beta-1a on MSFC progression in secondary progressive MS. *Neurology* 2002;59:679–87.

Comi G, Filippi M, Barkhof F et al.; Early Treatment of Multiple Sclerosis Study Group. Effect of early interferon treatment on conversion to definite multiple sclerosis: a randomised study. *Lancet* 2001;357:1576–82.

Comi G, Filippi M, Wolinsky JS; European/Canadian Glatiramer Acetate Study Group. The European/Canadian multicenter, double-blind, randomized, placebo-controlled study of the effects of glatiramer acetate on magnetic resonance imaging-measured disease activity and burden in patients with relapsing multiple sclerosis. *Ann Neurol* 2001;49:290–7.

Hartung HP, Gonsette R, Konig N et al. Mitoxantrone in progressive multiple sclerosis: a placebo-controlled, double-blind, randomised, multicentre trial. *Lancet* 2003;360:2018–25.

IFNβ Multiple Sclerosis Study Group and University of British Columbia MS/MRI Analysis Group. Interferon beta-1b in the treatment of multiple sclerosis: final outcome of the randomized controlled trial. *Neurology* 1995;45:1277–85.

Jacobs LD, Beck RW, Simon JH et al. Intramuscular interferon beta-1a therapy initiated during a first demyelinating event in multiple sclerosis. CHAMPS Study Group. *N Engl J Med* 2000;343:898–904.

Jacobs LD, Cookfair DL, Rudick RA et al. Intramuscular interferon beta-1a for disease progression in relapsing multiple sclerosis. The Multiple Sclerosis Collaborative Research Group (MSCRG). *Ann Neurol* 1996;39:285–94.

Johnson, KP, Brooks BR, Cohen J et al.; Copolymer 1 Multiple Sclerosis Study Group. Extended use of glatiramer acetate (Copaxone) is well tolerated and maintains its clinical effect on multiple sclerosis relapse rate and degree of disability. *Neurology* 1998;50:701–8.

Kappos L, Weinshenker B, Pozzilli C et al. Interferon beta-1b in secondary progressive MS: a combined analysis of the two trials. *Neurology* 2004;63:1779–87.

Leary SM, Miller DH, Stevenson VL et al. Interferon beta-1a in primary progressive MS: an exploratory, randomized, controlled trial. *Neurology* 2003;60:44–51.

Miller DH, Khan OA, Sheremata WA et al.; International Natalizumab Multiple Sclerosis Trial Group. A controlled trial of natalizumab for relapsing multiple sclerosis. *N Engl J Med* 2003;348:15–23.

Panitch H, Goodin DS, Francis G et al. Randomized, comparative study of interferon beta-1a treatment regimens in MS: The EVIDENCE Trial. *Neurology* 2002;59:1496–506.

PRISMS (Prevention of Relapses and Disability by Interferon beta-1a Subcutaneously in Multiple Sclerosis) Study Group. Randomised double-blind placebo-controlled study of interferon beta-1a in relapsing/remitting multiple sclerosis. *Lancet* 1998;352:1498–504; erratum 1999; 353:678.

SPECTRIMS (Secondary Progressive Efficacy Clinical Trial of Recombinant Interferon-beta-1a in MS) Study Group. Randomized controlled trial of interferon beta-1a in secondary progressive MS. Clinical results. *Neurology* 2001;56: 1496–504.

Wolinsky JS, Toyka KV, Kappos L, Grossberg SE. Interferon-beta antibodies: implications for the treatment of MS. *Lancet Neurol* 2003;2:528.

www.fda.gov/cder/foi/label/2004/ 125104lbl.pdf (natalizumab)

The role of paramedical staff and support groups

Doctors have become increasingly aware of the need to understand their patient's perception of their own lifestyle and of the measures that, through the intervention of paramedical staff, might be taken to enhance the patient's quality of life. A number of studies of quality of life among patients with multiple sclerosis (MS) have been performed. Although conclusions are difficult to draw from these appraisals (differing test formats have been applied), the patients have generally scored poorly in certain areas – particularly physical functioning and vitality – when compared with patients with other chronic diseases or healthy controls.

Attempts to modify the patient's level of disability can be considered either through inpatient rehabilitation or through concerted action by various paramedical staff on an outpatient basis.

Inpatient rehabilitation

Inpatient rehabilitation will usually be multidisciplinary. Healthcare professionals will aim to devise a program of therapy that fits the patient's needs and that is thoroughly understood and approved by the patient. The exact value of such rehabilitation remains uncertain, not least because of the various outcome measures used to measure the benefit of any intervention, and because of the multifactorial nature of the influences that might affect outcome.

Studies have suggested that patients with MS benefit from inpatient rehabilitation in various aspects of everyday life, including self-care activities, transfers and homemaking skills. These benefits are not simply confined to those patients showing a reduction in neurological impairment during the rehabilitation period. Analysis of the long-term nature of any benefit achieved during the inpatient rehabilitation period suggests it may well depend on the therapeutic input following discharge.

Community care

In both the UK and USA, the prevalence of MS is approximately 100 per 100 000; half of all patients with MS are estimated to be disabled. Disability, in this context, refers to any restriction or lack of ability to perform any activity of everyday living. Handicap is defined as a disadvantage, arising out of a particular disability, that limits or prevents an individual from performing a particular role in society. Although the individual contributions of the paramedical team are discussed below, their integration as a seamless service is of vital importance to the patient's welfare (Case history 7.1).

Case history 7.1 – the multidisciplinary team

A 45-year-old woman had had MS for 23 years. She had a partner and three children, the youngest of whom was 12 years old. Her partner had left his work in order to care for her, and was receiving appropriate benefits. He performed all the household tasks, carried out the shopping and attended to his partner's toilet and bath needs. The patient's 12-year-old daughter had recently been in trouble at school, with a poor disciplinary record and frequent truanting.

The patient's primary care provider organized a home visit by a multidisciplinary team based at the local hospital. The occupational therapists organized a number of aids for the patient, including a hoist and bath aids. The social worker organized attendance at a day center, arranged for carers to assist with everyday care, and organized a period of respite for the patient while her partner and their daughter had a holiday together. Finally, the social worker arranged for the couple's daughter to see a clinical psychologist.

Chronic neurological illness places a huge burden on the patient's family. Early intervention and the provision of appropriate support can go some way to preventing psychological distress in those caring for the patient.

Physiotherapist. The intervention of a physiotherapist is valuable in the assessment and treatment of spasticity, alongside drug therapy. Spasticity is enhanced by noxious stimuli from bladder infection, pressure sores or fecal impaction. Management of these problems alone can considerably reduce the level of spasticity or flexor spasms.

Stretch exercises on spastic muscles diminish spasticity for some hours after the therapy and, if performed regularly, will inhibit the development of flexor spasms (see Figure 5.1, page 55).

Management of ataxia is difficult. Measures can be taken to compensate for ataxia using visual and sensory guidance, although in many MS sufferers multifocal disability inhibits the use of such compensatory mechanisms. Regular input from the physiotherapist is valuable for refreshing techniques for the activities of daily living.

Occupational therapist. The occupational therapist is particularly involved in assessments of daily living, with a view to determining areas of difficulty and then seeking, by the use of modified techniques or aids, to improve function in that area and promote independence. The Barthel index is widely used in this context (Table 7.1). The index does not cover certain critical activities, for example cooking and communication, so additional test systems may be needed to obtain a full picture of the patient's disability.

Areas in which appliances may prove of value include adapted cutlery, and dressing and bathing aids. For more severely disabled patients, environmental control systems can maintain independence.

As walking deteriorates, various walking appliances can be introduced (Figure 7.1), culminating eventually in the use of a wheelchair. Choice of chair is critical and will be influenced by whether the chair is for indoor or outdoor use, whether any additional appliances need to be attached to the chair, and whether the chair is propelled by the patient, by a carer or electronically (Figure 7.2). Many disabled patients can continue to drive, provided they use an appropriately adapted car and have received instruction at a specialized assessment center (see Useful addresses, page 88).

TABLE 7.1

The modified Barthel index for activities of daily living

Bowels

0   Incontinent or needs enemas

1   Occasional accident

2   Continent

Bladder

0   Incontinent or catheterized

1   Occasional accident

2   Continent for > 7 successive days

Grooming

0   Needs help with personal care

1   Independent, with aids if necessary

Toilet use

0   Dependent

1   Needs some help

2   Fully independent

Feeding

0   Unable

1   Needs help

2   Independent

Transfers

0   Unable, no sitting balance

1   Major help (one or two people, physical); can sit

2   Minor help (verbal or physical)

3   Independent

Mobility

0   Immobile

1   Independent with wheelchair

2   Walks with help of one person

3   Independent, with aids if necessary

Dressing

0   Dependent

1   Needs help

2   Independent

Stairs

0   Unable

1   Needs help

2   Independent

Bathing

0   Dependent

1   Independent

Total

0–4	Very severely disabled
5–9	Severely disabled
10–14	Moderately disabled
15–19	Mildly disabled
20	Physically independent, but not necessarily normal or socially independent

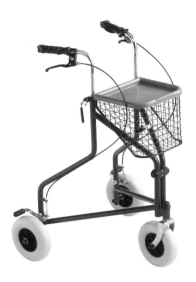

Figure 7.1 A walking frame can be used as walking ability declines. Reproduced with permission from Invacare Ltd.

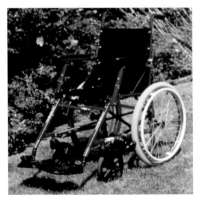

Figure 7.2 A wheelchair that collapses when not in use can be particularly convenient for patients who travel regularly. Reproduced with permission from Homecraft Rolyan Ltd, UK.

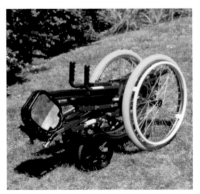

Speech and swallow therapists. Patients with MS may experience both dysarthria and dysphagia at some stage (Case history 7.2). Speech therapy may enable the patient to find various strategies to help compensate for a cerebellar dysarthria. Communication aids are only likely to help those patients with reasonably intact vision and upper-limb coordination (Figure 7.3).

Swallow function is best assessed by video fluoroscopy and analysis of the time it takes to swallow fluids and boluses of differing consistency. Sucking ice prior to eating may lessen bulbar spasticity, while altering posture during swallowing can reduce laryngeal penetration.

Social worker. The social worker, with the physician, can often provide a focus for the patient's ongoing care. In addition, the social

---

Case history 7.2 – dysphagia

A 60-year-old man had developed late-onset MS 6 years previously. He had experienced a progressive disability from the outset, and had exhibited bulbar symptoms for the previous 3 years. He tended to choke at times when swallowing, followed by bouts of violent coughing. He was admitted to hospital with evidence of a chest infection. Aspiration pneumonia was diagnosed.

The patient was referred to the speech and language therapists during his admission. When he had completely recovered, video fluoroscopy was performed, during which tracheal penetration was observed when the patient swallowed food of certain textures.

Following advice regarding swallow technique and use of foods of particular consistency, the patient's bouts of paroxysmal choking were considerably reduced.

Video fluoroscopy performed by a specialist speech and swallow therapist provides useful information about the nature of a patient's swallow problem, and may allow therapeutic intervention.

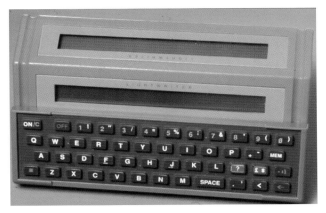

Figure 7.3 A communication aid. Reproduced with permission from Easiaids, UK.

worker is well placed to assess the effect of the patient's illness both on the patient and on the family unit. They are able to advise on financial matters, and can integrate any hospital care with the appropriate community services. Together with the occupational therapist, the social worker can advise on housing needs. Together with the family physician, the social worker can develop a care package for the more disabled patient. This will integrate various components of a home-support system and provide advice on the benefits of attendance at day centers that cater for patients with MS, or on the value of periodic inpatient stays linked with an active rehabilitation program.

Psychologist. Although it is often assumed that cognitive difficulties occur only in the later stages of MS, and then correlate with measures of physical disability, neither premise is correct. There is little correlation between cognitive impairment and disease duration, or with other measures of neurological impairment. Cognitive impairment is a predictor of handicap, and an indicator that the patient will eventually become dependent. Problems with abstract reasoning, memory and attention will interfere with the patient's understanding of their condition and their capacity to make decisions for the future. The potential to benefit from rehabilitation programs is likely to be correspondingly diminished.

Besides an assessment of intellectual function, the psychologist may well need to assist the patient's emotional adjustment to the initial diagnosis and the subsequent effects of the disease.

Specialist nurse. Specialist nurses with a particular interest and expertise in one aspect of neurological disability can now be found working in fields such as MS, epilepsy and Parkinson's disease. A specialist nurse can fulfill several roles, including:
- input following initial diagnosis
- discussion of care (including the use of new drugs) with the patient
- liaison with the family physician and the hospital service as new needs are identified.

Patient support groups. The UK's MS Society, and the National Multiple Sclerosis Society and its many chapters in the USA, provide a valuable resource of information and guidance (see Useful addresses, pages 87 and 89). They offer objective advice on the many issues relating to the disease, for example in relation to diet or the role of disease-modifying therapy, and discussion on the various symptoms encountered by patients. Patients can receive advice on benefits and on local networks of the society, which can then provide support on a 'one-to-one' basis.

The Disabled Living Foundation serves as a source of information for patients with disabilities, and for those professional staff dealing with them (see Useful addresses, page 87). The foundation has a reference library and a comprehensive information service. Over 30 Disabled Living Centres have been established in the UK, where patients can try out a variety of aids, backed, in most instances, by expert advice. In addition, the centers hold meetings and study days to broaden knowledge among care workers and concerned individuals dealing with people with MS or other conditions associated with long-term disability.

Key points – the role of paramedical staff and support groups

- A multidisciplinary approach is vital when considering the needs of patients with more advanced MS.
- Occasional periods of inpatient rehabilitation are of proven value in patients with MS.
- Regular physiotherapy reduces the liability to develop flexor spasms.
- Occupational therapy is of particular value in identifying the patient's home needs.
- Support organizations for MS can give valuable support to patients and their families.

Key references

Francabandera FL, Holland NJ, Wiesel-Levison P, Scheinberg LC. Multiple sclerosis rehabilitation: inpatient vs. outpatient. *Rehabil Nurs* 1988;13:251–3.

Fuller KJ, Dawson K, Wiles CM. Physiotherapy in chronic multiple sclerosis: a controlled trial. *Clin Rehabil* 1996;10:195–204.

Kirker SGB, Young E, Warlow CP. An evaluation of a multiple sclerosis liaison nurse. *Clin Rehabil* 1995;9: 219–26.

Mertin J. Rehabilitation in multiple sclerosis. *Ann Neurol* 1994; 36(suppl):S130–3.

Thompson AJ, Johnston S, Harrison J et al. Service delivery in multiple sclerosis: the need for coordinated community care. *MS Management* 1997;4:11–21.

Advances in both basic and applied research into multiple sclerosis (MS) over the past few decades have been substantial, and the application of new investigative techniques promises to further shape our understanding of this disease, which has for so long been considered enigmatic.

Etiology

Immune-mediated response. Available data confirm there is an immunopathogenic component to the disease process of MS. It is difficult to determine whether the immune mechanisms are a primary part of the pathogenesis or reflect a response to a persistent central nervous system (CNS) infection in which nervous system tissue is damaged secondarily by an otherwise well-directed immune response. The continued application of modern molecular techniques should establish the importance of any persistent CNS infection in directing a secondary immunopathogenic response. It may well be that the development of more specific and effective immuno-modulatory therapies will disprove the theory that incomplete responses to such treatments are due to persistent CNS infection.

Genetic profile. Several independent studies to identify the genetic profiles for disease susceptibility in members of multiplex MS families have been somewhat disappointing. It is likely, however, that a considerable proportion of the clinical phenotypic variation common in MS will be explained by the genotypes that control patterns of immune expression at the cellular level, such as the proportions and amounts of chemokines and cytokines secreted on immune activation. These profiles may help clinicians to better characterize the different disease phenotypes early on, that is, help to identify monophasic demyelinating diseases, relapsing forms of MS associated with little acquired disability over decades, rapidly progressive forms of MS, and perhaps primary progressive disease.

Diagnosis and disease staging

Magnetic resonance imaging (MRI) has contributed substantially to our understanding of the dynamics of the disease process, and is now incorporated into the diagnostic criteria for MS (see Chapter 4, page 43). Certain patterns observed on cerebral and spinal MRI scans may allow MS to be more rapidly diagnosed before the patient experiences classic recurrent clinical attacks, thereby providing better short-term prognostic precision. However, clinicians still need better information to understand the disease in patients who have clinically definite and laboratory-supported MS but in whom neuroimaging scans of the entire neural axis are normal.

Therapy

As more sophisticated imaging approaches are introduced into clinical practice, including the more routine use of magnetic resonance (MR) spectroscopic imaging and other advanced MR techniques, imaging profiles specific to biologically meaningful clinical disease phenotypes and genotypes, with both prognostic and therapeutic implications, are likely to emerge.

Clinicians may also be able to recognize an increasing number of MRI signatures of the effects of different drugs, such as the profound early effects of interferons and natalizumab on enhancement, or the delayed effect of glatiramer on the evolution of late tissue destruction in evolving lesions. Differences in both the apparent mechanisms of action and the MRI signatures of various new immunomodulatory agents may allow for the rational choice of drugs for individual patients, and for the informed study of combined therapies.

As the systemic inflammatory component of new lesion formation comes under increasing control with the current generation of immunomodulators, attention should shift to the development and application of neuroprotectants designed to readily penetrate the CNS and to improve axonal integrity and neuronal survival.

It is also possible that our new knowledge of antibody-stimulated remyelination will lead to the discovery of effective small-peptide ligands that stimulate oligodendroglial-cell regeneration, ushering in therapeutic trials with an endpoint of clinical improvement, rather than slowing disease progression.

Key references

Barkhof F, Rocca M, Francis G et al.; Early Treatment of Multiple Sclerosis Study Group. Validation of diagnostic magnetic resonance imaging criteria for multiple sclerosis and response to interferon beta1a. *Ann Neurol* 2003;53:718–24.

Frohman EM, Goodin DS, Calabresi PA et al. The utility of MRI in suspected MS: report of the Therapeutics and Technology Assessment Subcommittee of the American Academy of Neurology. *Neurology* 2003;61:602–11.

Sturzebecher S, Wandinger KP, Rosenwald A et al. Expression profiling identifies responder and non-responder phenotypes to interferon-beta in multiple sclerosis. *Brain* 2003;126:1419–29.

Useful addresses

UK

The MS Society
372 Edgware Road
London NW2 6ND
Tel: +44 (0)20 8438 0700
Helpline: 0808 800 8000
www.mssociety.org.uk

Multiple Sclerosis Trust
Spirella Building, Bridge Road
Letchworth Garden City
Herts SG6 4ET
Tel: +44 (0)1462 476700
Fax: +44 (0)1462 476710
info@mstrust.org.uk
www.mstrust.org.uk

College of Occupational Therapists
106–114 Borough High Street
London SE1 1LB
Tel: +44 (0)20 7357 6480
www.cot.co.uk

The Chartered Society of Physiotherapy
14 Bedford Row
London WC1R 4ED
Tel: +44 (0)20 7306 6666
Fax: +44 (0)20 7306 6611
www.csp.org.uk

Carers UK
20–25 Glasshouse Yard
London EC1A 4JT
Tel: +44 (0)20 7490 8818
Fax: +44 (0)20 7490 8824
Carers Line: 0808 808 7777
(Weds/Thurs 10 AM–12 PM and
2 PM–4 PM)
info@carersuk.org
www.carersuk.org

Connect
16–18 Marshalsea Road
London SE1 1HL
Tel: +44 (0)20 7367 0840
Fax: +44 (0)20 7367 0841
info@ukconnect.org
www.ukconnect.org

Disabled Living Foundation
380–384 Harrow Road
London W9 2HU
Tel: +44 (0)20 7289 6111
Helpline: 0845 130 9177
(Mon–Fri 10 AM–4 PM)
info@dlf.org.uk
www.dlf.org.uk

DIAL UK (The National Association of Disablement Information and Advice Lines)
St Catherine's
Tickhill Road
Doncaster DN4 8QN
Tel: +44 (0)1302 310123
Fax: +44 (0)1302 310404
enquiries@dialuk.org.uk
www.dialuk.org.uk

Royal Association for Disability and Rehabilitation
12 City Forum
250 City Road
London EC1V 8AF
Tel: +44 (0)20 7250 3222
Fax: +44 (0)20 7250 0212
radar@radar.org.uk
www.radar.org.uk

Speakability
1 Royal Street
London SE1 7LL
Tel: +44 (0)20 7261 9572
Fax: +44 (0)20 7928 9542
Helpline: 0808 808 9572
(Mon–Fri 10 AM–4 PM)
speakability@speakability.org.uk
www.speakability.org.uk

Disability Scotland
Princess House
5 Shandwick Place
Edinburgh EH2 4RG
Tel: +44 (0)131 229 8632

Capability Scotland
11 Ellersly Road
Edinburgh EH12 6HY
Tel: +44 (0)131 313 5510
Fax: +44 (0)131 346 1681
ascs@capability-scotland.org.uk
www.capability-scotland.org.uk

Disability Wales
Wernddu Court
Caerphilly Business Park
Van Road
Caerphilly CF83 3ED
Tel: +44 (0)29 2088 7325
Fax: +44 (0)29 2088 8702
info@dwac.demon.co.uk
www.disabilitywales.org

Forum of Mobility Centres
(a network of 17 independent organizations in the UK that offer professional advice and assessment for individuals who have a medical condition or injury that may affect their ability to drive)
PO Box 883
Bradford BD8 0WX
Helpline: 0800 559 3636
(Mon–Fri 9 AM–5 PM)
enquiry@mobility-centres.org.uk
www.mobility-centres.org.uk

USA

National Multiple Sclerosis Society

(provides addresses of individual NMSS chapters and clinics, plus a variety of topical and updated information)
733 Third Avenue, 6th Floor
New York, NY 10017
Tel: +1 212 986 3240
Fax: +1 212 986 7981
Toll-free: 1 800 344 4867
info@nmss.org
www.nmss.org

Consortium of Multiple Sclerosis Centers

(includes an annotated list of member MS clinics and other useful information)
c/o Gimbel MS Center
718 Teaneck Road
Teaneck, NJ 07666
Tel: +1 201 837 0727
Fax: +1 201 837 9414
info@mscare.org
www.mscare.org

International

Multiple Sclerosis Australia

Studdy MS Center, Joseph Street
Lidcombe, NSW 2141
Tel: +61 (0)2 9646 0600
Fax: +61 (0)2 9646 0675
infoline@mssociety.com.au
www.msaustralia.org.au

Multiple Sclerosis Society of Canada

175 Bloor Street East
Suite 700, North Tower
Toronto, Ontario M4W 3R8
Tel: +1 416 922 6065
Fax: +1 416 922 7538
Toll-free: 1 800 268 7582
info@mssociety.ca (provide your town/province in your e-mail)
www.mssociety.ca

Multiple Sclerosis International Federation

(registration on this site provides automatic weekly alerts to new information or patient correspondence and provides links to the websites of all major national MS societies)
3rd Floor Skyline House
200 Union Street
London SE1 0LX
Tel: +44 (0)20 7620 1911
Fax: +44 (0)20 7620 1922
info@msif.org
www.msif.org

Index

What the reviewers say:

This book is a little goldmine and
is very good value for money

On *Fast Facts – Endometriosis, 2nd edn*, in *Medical Journal of Australia*, 2004

concise and well written and accompanied by numerous excellent color
illustrations... an excellent little book! Score: 100 - 5 Stars

On *Fast Facts – Sexual Dysfunction*
in *Doody's Health Sciences Review*, 2004

pleasingly pithy, erudite and accessible,
as well as being helpfully informative

On *Fast Facts – Bipolar Disorder, 2nd edn*, in *Medical Journal of Australia*, 2004

a timely and accessible book...
a worthwhile and handy tool for medical students

On *Fast Facts – Dyspepsia*, in *Digestive and Liver Disease 36*, 2004

provides a lot of information in a concise and easily accessible format...
a practical guide to managing most lower respiratory tract infections

On *Fast Facts – Respiratory Tract Infection*,
in *Respiratory Care* 49(1), 2004

an invaluable guide
to the latest thinking

On *Fast Facts – Irritable Bowel Syndrome*, in *Update*, 4 September 2003

a rapid guide to understanding dementia...
value for money and I would definitely recommend it

On *Fast Facts – Dementia*, in *South African Medical Journal* 93(10), 2003

an extremely useful guide

On *Fast Facts – Psoriasis*, 2nd edn,
in *Clinical and Experimental Dermatology*, 2005

will likely be read cover to cover in just one or
two sittings by all who are fortunate enough
to obtain a copy

On *Fast Facts – Benign Prostatic Hyperplasia*, 4th edn, in *Doody's Health Sciences Review*, Dec 2002

explains the important facts and demonstrates
the levels of "good practice" that can be achieved

On *Fast Facts – Minor Surgery*,
in *Journal of the Royal Society for the Promotion of Health* 122(3), 2002

a splendid publication

On *Fast Facts – Sexually Transmitted Infections*, in *Journal of Antimicrobial Chemotherapy* 49, 2002

I enthusiastically recommend this
stimulating, short book which should
be required reading for all clinicians

On *Fast Facts – Irritable Bowel Syndrome*, in *Gastroenterology* 120(6), 2001

the style is succinct and the included material is current, clinically
relevant, focused, and designed for easy availability

On *Fast Facts – Chronic Obstructive Pulmonary Disease*,
in *Respiratory Care*, Jan 2005

quite simply,
a terrific little book

On *Fast Facts – Smoking Cessation*, in *Medical Journal of Australia*, Jun 2005

www.fastfacts.com

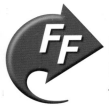

Imagine
if every time you wanted
to know something you
knew where to look...

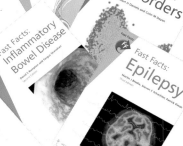

Over one million copies sold

- Written by world experts
- Concise and practical
- Up to date
- Designed for ease of reading and reference
- Copiously illustrated with useful photographs,
  diagrams and charts.

Our aim for *Fast Facts* is to be **the world's most respected medical
handbook series**. Feedback on how to make titles even more useful is
always welcome (feedback@fastfacts.com).

Over 70 *Fast Facts* titles, including:

Allergic Rhinitis
Asthma
Benign Gynecological Disease (second edition)
Benign Prostatic Hyperplasia (fifth edition)
Bipolar Disorder
Bladder Cancer
Bleeding Disorders
Brain Tumors
Breast Cancer (third edition)
Celiac Disease
Chronic Obstructive Pulmonary Disease
Colorectal Cancer (second edition)
Contraception (second edition)
Dementia
Depression (second edition)
Dyspepsia (second edition)
Eczema and Contact Dermatitis
Endometriosis (second edition)
Epilepsy (third edition)
Erectile Dysfunction (third edition)
Gynecological Oncology

Headaches (second edition)
Hyperlipidemia (third edition)
Hypertension (second edition)
Inflammatory Bowel Disease
Irritable Bowel Syndrome (second edition)
Menopause (second edition)
Minor Surgery
Osteoporosis (fourth edition)
Parkinson's Disease
Prostate Cancer (fourth edition)
Psoriasis (second edition)
Respiratory Tract Infection (second edition)
Rheumatoid Arthritis
Schizophrenia (second edition)
Sexual Dysfunction
Sexually Transmitted Infections
Skin Cancer
Smoking Cessation
Soft Tissue Rheumatology
Thyroid Disorders
Urinary Stones

Orders

To order via the website, or to find regional distributors,
please go to www.fastfacts.com

For telephone orders, please call +44 (0)1752 202301 (Europe),
1 800 247 6553 (USA, toll free) or +1 419 281 1802 (Americas)